Ethics in an Epidemic

Ethics in an Epidemic

AIDS, Morality, and Culture

Timothy F. Murphy

UNIVERSITY OF CALIFORNIA PRESS

Berkeley / Los Angeles / London

University of California Press
Berkeley and Los Angeles, California

University of California Press
London, England

Copyright © 1994 by The Regents of the University of California

Library of Congress Cataloging-in-Publication Data
Murphy, Timothy F., 1954–
    Ethics in an epidemic : AIDS, morality, and culture / Timothy
F. Murphy.
        p.   cm.
    Includes bibliographical references and index.
    ISBN 0–520–08636–8 (alk. paper)
    1. AIDS (Disease)—Moral and ethical aspects.   2. AIDS
(Disease)—Social aspects.   3. AIDS (Disease)—Government
policy—United States.   I. Title.
RA644.A25M87   1994
362.1'969792—dc20   94-8248
                                                          CIP

Printed in the United States of America

1   2   3   4   5   6   7   8   9

The paper used in this publication meets the minimum requirements of
American National Standard for Information Sciences—Permanence of
Paper for Printed Library Materials, ANSI Z39.48-1984 ⊚

Contents

ACKNOWLEDGMENTS   vii

Introduction   1

PART ONE: THE MEANING OF AIDS

1
The Once and Future Epidemic   11

2
The Search for a Cure   28

3
Testimony   52

PART TWO: HIV TESTING

4
Celebrities and AIDS   69

5
The Angry Death of Kimberly Bergalis   82

6
Health-Care Workers with HIV   93

7
Teaching AIDS in China   108

PART THREE: AIDS POLITICS

8
HIV at the Borders   129

9
Politics and Priorities   144

10
No Time for an AIDS Backlash   162

Afterword   183

NOTES   189

INDEX   213

Acknowledgments

I wish to thank the following people for advice I much appreciated during the writing of the various parts of this book: Jerry McCarthy, Richard D. Mohr, Sheryl Stevenson, and Thomas Dukes. I especially want to thank my University of Illinois College of Medicine colleagues Norman Gevitz, Marc Lappé, Suzanne Poirier, and Barbara F. Sharf for their counsel as they read and commented on early sections of the manuscript. I wish to express my gratitude to Amanda Frost for her assiduous editing of the manuscript. I also much value University of California Press sponsoring editor Elizabeth Knoll's sustained interest across the years that rolled away between the original idea for this book and its actual advent. Lastly, I want to acknowledge David E. Tolman, M.D., with whom I had my very first conversations about AIDS long ago in simpler times at the Chateau Din.

Introduction

For varied and complex reasons the HIV/AIDS epidemic continues to insinuate itself into the fabric of contemporary life not only in this nation but across the world. So pervasive is the epidemic that it appears that the great chain of being is held together by a virus. But because human lives and futures are amenable to choice, we are not mere onlookers to an ineluctable advance of the epidemic. Moral philosophy began when human beings found themselves free from the predestination of biological imperative and discovered the necessity of confronting their fates as in part a matter of their own choosing. Ethics is an amalgam of different kinds of analyses and inquiries whose goal is the identification and pursuit of the goals that ennoble human life and spare it from degradation and whose value is that of wisdom. Ethics is both the rapture and burden of human choice.

Ethical disputes about the Acquired Immune Deficiency Syndrome (AIDS) and its causal agents, the family of Human Immunodeficiency Viruses (HIV), are conducted in the brusque discourse of everyday life, in the headlines of the tabloids, and in the more forbidding argot of medical researchers and academic scholars. A cascade of disputes has dogged the epidemic from the beginning. Certain questions appear to have come and gone: Is some kind of general quarantine necessary to protect the public health? Do indeterminacies of HIV testing undermine the morality of its use? Should gay men refrain from donating blood? Should bathhouses be seen as epicenters of infection and closed outright or should they be used as venues for education, education that might not otherwise occur? But the vacuum left here has only been filled by other questions. More recent questions about AIDS and ethics quite often involve the form and scope of HIV testing and the extent to which government ought to fund AIDS research and treatment. Other questions concern the status of people with HIV in employment and society. Can HIV infection, for example, count as a substantive reason for the exclusion of gay men and lesbians generally from open service in the U.S. military?[1] The range and scope of these questions is often overwhelming because of their magnitude, and the emotion they elicit is even more striking.

Unfortunately, impediments to a full appreciation of the importance of the epidemic and the questions it raises still exist. Knowing this, I probably should not have been surprised when a prominent philosopher asked if my work on this book about the epidemic reflected the latest trend. Far from being "trendy," the problems of the AIDS epidemic embody issues profoundly important to moral philosophy. Indeed, it is hard to think of a single question of bioethics that goes unraised by AIDS, that is not deepened by AIDS, even if some ethicists are fond of pointing out that AIDS does not raise any wholly novel questions. There are questions of informed consent in experimental trials, questions of the design of those trials, questions of the treatment of persons with AIDS (PWAs) at the deathbed, questions of contraception and abortion for women infected with HIV, questions of resource allocation, the design of the health-care system, and the professional responsibilities of health-care professionals who care for patients with HIV. The culture of AIDS, unfolding right before our eyes, recapitulates bioethics and many of the important questions that engage contemporary political and social theory as well.

AIDS took the United States by surprise as it precipitated novel, lethal syndromes at first largely in gay men and persons using needle-injected drugs. That initial epidemiology invited widely divergent social and moral interpretations of the epidemic. By reason of the issues it continues to raise starkly, AIDS is positioned at the juncture of critical debates about the nature of sexual morality and the limits of public authority. Involving sex, needles, bodily fluids, and unclosetings, AIDS has proved a motherlode for tabloid scandal and shock television. Involving language and representations, AIDS has become a battleground for the control of words and images, a battle over the very meaning of the epidemic. In addition, biomedical uncertainty about the epidemic invites speculation about causes, cures, and the morbidity of sexuality. Some have seen the epidemic as the punishment of a vengeful God. There have even been theories describing AIDS as the result of a deliberate conspiracy to rid the nation of "undesirables" by a "bioweapon attack."[2] More sophisticated though hardly less controversial analyses have argued for biomedical complicity in the origins of the epidemic, for example, claiming that programs of oral polio vaccination in Africa introduced pathogenic viruses into human populations.[3] Quacks have lured the hopeful and the hopeless into spending money on the most outlandish treatments: hydrogen peroxide injections, the food preservative butylated hydroxytoluene, herbal capsules containing toxic metals, and even pills derived from HIV-infected mice.[4] And the association of AIDS with gay sex, drug use, and prostitution has invoked powerful cultural and moral responses not only about control of the epidemic but even about how it should be discussed publicly.

There is no dearth of material for the moral philosopher here; no apology is needed for caring about an issue as important as the sickness and death of gay men, drug-users, their sexual partners, and their children. No apology is needed for trying to understand the ethical challenge of the epidemic even when its questions—for example, "Should Olympic athletes be tested for HIV infection?"—do not have a hoary, ivy-covered lineage. For all the very real and abiding damage the epidemic has left in its wake, if attention to the epidemic needs another justification than the care and cure of PWAs, AIDS has been and remains an unparalleled opportunity for moral reflection on the meaning of disease, the nature of the health-care system, the responsibilities of government, the uses of the law, and the relationship between conscience and activism.

In a short, posthumously published essay Friedrich Nietzsche asked

What, then is truth? A mobile army of metaphors, metonyms, and anthropomorphisms—in short, a sum of human relations, which have been enhanced, transposed, and embellished poetically and rhetorically, and which after long use seem firm, canonical, and obligatory to a people: truths are illusions about which one has forgotten that this is what they are: metaphors, which are worn out and without sensuous powers; coins which have lost their pictures, and now matter only as metal, no longer as coins.[5]

The "truths" of AIDS are often like the truths Nietzsche would unmask. Often posed as objective, detached assessments, the "truths" about AIDS carry with them marks of their own allegiance and empire. The "spread of AIDS," the "protection of the public health," the "foreign threat of AIDS," the "social impact of AIDS," all bear moral imprints that interpret the epidemic even as they "describe" it. Any analysis of AIDS must therefore consider not only the official "truths" but also the moral and cultural preconditions that make those "truths" possible.

Nietzsche saw, as none before him, that moral philosophy was finally as much about power as about the good. There is a point in moral philosophy where argument becomes rhetoric, where dialogue becomes strategy and discourse becomes domination. What is often at stake in the debates about the epidemic is usually much more than a particular decision about whether, for example, to resuscitate a particular gay man suffering cardiopulmonary arrest or whether sufficient evidence exists to make a particular drug available for prescription use. The moral debates in the HIV epidemic ultimately involve judgments and assumptions about the power of public and moral authority. They ultimately involve the power to name villains and heroes. They are finally about nothing less than the power to define moral reality.

The AIDS epidemic has thrown any number of such moral struggles into bold relief. Is AIDS the inevitable consequence of sexual and narcotic promiscuity and for that reason the punishment of God?[6] Or is it a crucible for the improvement of the human community? For example, Elisabeth Kübler-Ross has argued that the AIDS epidemic will turn out to be "the biggest and best teacher" of the essentials of human life, the worth of sharing, and acceptance of other human beings, regardless of color, creed, or sexual preference.[7] Mary Catherine Bateson and Richard Goldsby also connect AIDS to ultimate moral solutions:

The epidemic is a moment of opportunity for discovering the full potential of humanness. If we can use the impetus of AIDS to expand and apply knowledge cooperatively and humanely, we may also learn to control the dangers of the arms race and of world hunger and environmental degradation, for the imagination of AIDS is the imagination of human unity, intimately held in the interdependent web of life.[8]

But such analyses are not merely descriptions. These interpretations not only explain, they also *advance a cause.*

What may be expected from moral analysis of the AIDS epidemic which self-consciously acknowledges its own directive nature? By its very nature moral knowledge, and moral self-knowledge especially, is always and necessarily incomplete. We are, after all, finite beings and self-forgiving beings at that. Where there is incompleteness, there is room for indeterminacy and a plurality of competing moral views. For reasons that belong to the nature of human knowledge, psychology, and culture, it is not surprising that people have come to competing moral interpretations of the AIDS epidemic and its "solutions." Any moral analysis is ultimately a confession of values thought to define the worth and integrity of human life. In this book I try to look at a number of issues that deserve special consideration at this moment in this nation's epidemic. By looking at these issues I will have done only what each individual must eventually do: name the goods and goals that he or she thinks best serve the worth and dignity of human beings because of the experience they bring, the lessons they teach, the values they serve, and the legacy they leave behind. What I try to do here is point out ways in which not AIDS per se but its cultural and moral interpretation frame many of the assessments of the nature of the epidemic and what responses are thereby thought appropriate.

In part 1 I consider the way the moral significance of AIDS has been represented in histories of the epidemic, social commentaries, cinematic representations, narratives about the search for an AIDS cure, and obituaries. In the first chapter of this section, "The Once and Future Epidemic," I look at how accounts of the origins and history of the epidemic often locate the blame for the epidemic on individual gay men or gay values in general. Commentaries about the future of the epidemic tip their moral hand inasmuch as they often declaim the social damages of AIDS while simultaneously exiling those damages to years yet to come. These foretellings, darkening the present with a future parade of horribles, are therefore free to advance moral conclusions about the nature of public authority and sexual morality without fear of contradiction. While expectations about the future of the epidemic function to divert attention from its present effects, they also paradoxically sustain and distend the hope of PWAs whose hope is never far from anguish in regard to a treatment or cure. In "The Search for a Cure" I argue that expectations about the workings of medicine, despite their significance as emblems of human progress, sometimes ironically open PWAs to new throes of hopelessness. Medicine can frustrate the hopes of individual PWAs because even the most theoretically sophisticated experiments can fail and because the values of medicine may foster false hope, homophobia, and dehumanizing treatment. The third chapter in this section, "Testimony," looks at the writing about those who have not survived the epidemic. While criticism has been directed at elegiac responses to the epidemic, this chapter advances the view that the blessing of the dead that appears in obituaries, memorials, and the Names Project Quilt is an important part of the moral response to the epidemic. Elegies need not be mere keening, and keening need not be dismissed so readily since the term also means a call for vengeance against wrongful death and so raises its own moral imperatives. We are not surprised then that testimony about the dead is often continuous with exhortations to political and social activism against the epidemic. Passing over the dead in silence would be as much an abrogation of moral responsibility in the epidemic as failing to protest any policy that permits continued, inadvertent HIV infection.

The chapters of part 2 explore a number of questions related to policies about and advocacy of HIV testing, especially the view that widespread HIV testing is an essential component for the control of the epidemic. A letter from the *New England Journal of Medicine,* discussed in "Celebrities and AIDS," promotes exactly such a view when it argues for public disclosure by celebrities about the diagnosis of HIV/AIDS and the physician's responsibility to solicit such disclosure. Using data from an HIV test site in California, this letter correlates HIV testing with disclosures about the rich and famous with AIDS, noting how celebrity disclosures significantly increase requests for HIV testing. But the extent to which HIV testing depends on celebrity disclosures may be understood as evidence of social failure in educating the public about the nature of HIV risks and the significance of HIV testing. Reliance on celebrity disclosures can only prove an occasional benefit to larger educational and health-care objectives. The question of HIV testing is also worth considering not only in relation to the public but also in regard to health-care professionals. Following the discovery that Kimberly Bergalis's infection with HIV occurred during dental treatment, she and her family committed themselves to the cause of HIV testing for all health-care workers. "The Angry Death of Kimberly Bergalis" offers an argument for the wastefulness of such testing and an explanation for the appeal of universal, mandatory, continuous testing: the perception that AIDS is "leaking" from the risk groups of gay men and drug-users. Far from being an issue of medical safety, reaction to Bergalis's highly unusual infection signifies the fears and authoritarian propensities of a public that does not otherwise see itself at risk of HIV infection. The next chapter, "Health-Care Workers with HIV," carries out a sustained analysis of the question of whether health-care workers have the duty to disclose their own HIV and AIDS diagnoses to patients under their care. I argue that there is no convincing moral argument to sustain such a view under all circumstances: a patient's wish to know about HIV infection in a health-care worker is an insufficient warrant for compelled disclosure given the typically limited risk of infection and the absence of required disclosures in other areas of similar risk. The question of HIV testing of health-care workers also figured in my instructional responsibilities in a course on leadership and ethics taught in 1992 at the Beijing Medical University in the People's Republic of China. In that course I described the epidemic in the United States to a class of physicians and other health-care professionals and asked them in one assignment to formulate policy on HIV-infected health workers for a hypothetical hospital in their country. I report their reactions, their proposals, and my experience on a University of Illinois committee charged to formulate policy of exactly that kind in "Teaching AIDS in China." I was not surprised that certain assumptions that guided U.S. reaction in the early epidemic reappeared in the Chinese students' thinking about the moral causality and infectivity of AIDS, the widely divergent political and cultural systems of the two nations notwithstanding.

The last section of the book, part 3—AIDS Politics, considers certain AIDS issues that bear on political questions in the United States, especially those related to the civil rights of people with HIV. The first chapter of this section, "HIV at the Borders," assesses U.S. policies on the entrance to this country of foreign nationals infected with HIV. In contrast to its self-assured and self-imposed ideal as the world's refuge from tyrannies of many kinds, U.S. policy on HIV not only proves prejudicial toward people with HIV but is inconsistent with its policy declarations elsewhere on civil rights. Furthermore, the current policy is not well substantiated by the two main arguments typically used in its defense: protecting the public health and protecting the taxpayer's wallet. The issue of foreign nationals with HIV was prominent in the 1992 presidential campaign (and after), and the chapter "Politics and Priorities" assesses the way in which presidential candidates proposed governmental action on AIDS matters. While all three main presidential candidates (George Bush, Bill Clinton, and Ross Perot) saw the need for government action against the epidemic, none was willing to assume the mantle of AIDS activist. The last section of that chapter also considers a 1993 report from the National Research Council about the status of the epidemic. That report, while ostensibly arguing that AIDS will not have the kind of dire social consequences announced during the previous decade, has the effect of burying the epidemic under already existing social problems. It announces the banality of AIDS. What social obligations are there then in regard to the epidemic? The last chapter, "No

Time for an AIDS Backlash," critically assesses claims that society has already met or exceeded its responsibilities toward AIDS education, prevention, treatment, and research. While it is indeed difficult to set priorities in an age of moral pluralism and finite resources, there is no good reason to think that enough has already been done to foil the epidemic and to help those affected by it.

Art critic and AIDS activist Douglas Crimp has observed that "AIDS does not exist apart from the practices that conceptualize it, represent it, and respond to it. We know AIDS only in and through those practices."[9] To be sure, AIDS is not only about the microbiological facts of HIV. Although HIV infection and its illnesses are as important to immunology as to moral and social analysis, the debates about AIDS are taking place in social contexts in which larger moral battles are being waged: about the conduct of sexual life, the allocation of health-care services and other social goods, the authority of government, and the ethics of representations in the media, literature, and elsewhere. We cannot therefore expect the dilemmas of the epidemic to be completely, finally resolved in contexts where larger issues are themselves in dispute. For that reason I surely do not pretend to have "solved" every moral dilemma of the epidemic, especially when knowledge about the epidemic and its social significance are still in flux. Finally, I must also acknowledge that my study is limited further to the extent that it focuses mostly on AIDS in the United States. I hope nonetheless to have resisted certain facile and morally invidious analyses of the epidemic which permit self-serving moral interpretations, reckless public responses, wasteful public policies, homophobia, and the social and moral invisibility of PWAs, this in order to identify ways in which liberty, dignity, the plenitude of moral being, and hope properly constituted can be preserved and nurtured even under the shadow of the epidemic.

PART ONE

The Meaning of AIDS

1

The Once and Future Epidemic

In *And the Band Played On* gay journalist Randy Shilts introduces one of the figures central to his history of the origins of the AIDS epidemic—Gaetan Dugas—at the 1980 San Francisco gay pride parade: Dugas's diagnosis of Kaposi's sarcoma just a few weeks before had not dampened his spirits since he expected the blemishes to disappear.[1] In the pages that follow, Shilts paints a picture of a self-absorbed profligate from whom AIDS radiated outward in an expanding circle, whose vainglorious sexuality enclosed others in the involuntary grip of AIDS. Mostly through *And the Band Played On* Dugas became known as "Patient Zero," the man whose erotic penchants and compulsions put him causally at ground zero of the American AIDS epidemic.[2] Shilts's portrait of Dugas recalls the literary visions of "anointers" who in earlier times "spread" bubonic plague,[3] and mass-media reports were quick to pick up the Dugas story in their headlines. Indeed, even the publisher's press release noted Dugas's story as one of the most salient features of the book.[4]

Others have also tried their hand at identifying the various forces that made the epidemic possible,[5] but *And the Band Played On* remains the most ambitious account thus far about the origins of the epidemic, about what persons and circumstances were responsible for the emergence of the unprecedented syndrome. And if there have been discussions about the origins of the epidemic, there have also been discussions about its future. In often dire and foreboding language many of these discussions conjure a future despoiled not only of health by the epidemic. Public health analyst Ronald Bayer's *Private Acts, Social Consequences: AIDS and the Politics of Public Health,* for example, summons a future beset by trials of immense consequence and gravity in matters of civil rights should progress against the epidemic not keep pace with public expectation.[6] In law professor Monroe Price's *Shattered Mirrors* there is also augury of a future fatalistically vulnerable to moral desperation and political derangement.[7] Part of Price's haruspicy here is achieved through word choice. The following words, for example, occur on a single page of *Shattered Mirrors* chosen at random: enemy, virus, bacteria, parasites, vulnerable, puzzle, change, pessimism, AIDS, unrelenting, mocking, resistant, microbes, quarantine, illness, incubated, infectious, poor, disgrace, unchecked, infection, problem, doubtful, competition, survival.[8] The connotative force of page after page of dire language of this kind suggests a viral cataclysm whose outcome will determine the moral and medical perfectibility of man.[9]

The description of a figure who "spreads" AIDS is worth conjoining with considerations about the future of AIDS for what the conjunction reveals about the way responsibility is understood and assigned in the AIDS epidemic, about the way we think of the epidemic as a catastrophe, and about what remedies it requires. Its future turns out to be even more problematic than its present.

The "Spread" of AIDS

In describing the figure central to his account Shilts describes Dugas as "ideal for this community," the pretty-boy gay community, that is, by virtue of his sandy hair, inviting smile, trendy Paris and London clothes, and soft Quebec accent. By Shilts's account Dugas lived a life of parties, cocaine, Quaaludes, bars, baths, "poppers" (amyl nitrate), and travel. Once "the major sissy of his neighborhood in Quebec City," Dugas was an ugly duckling who became a swan, who could say with confidence: "I am the prettiest one."[10] But his dangerous sexual liaisons, not his looks, earned Dugas prominence in Shilts's account. Dugas kept, for example, an address book that amounted to an archeological record of his sexual history, with strata so old that he sometimes did not recall the fossilized names he unearthed there. He was unapologetic about his wide circle of lovers, an erotic life all the more attractive to him—according to Shilts—as emotional compensation for an unhappy childhood. After years of taunting and torment by neighborhood bullies, he had carved "his own niche in the royalty of gay beauty, as a star of the homosexual jet set."[11] Dugas's mortal sin in Shilts's account was his unwillingness to abdicate his eminence in gay erotic hierarchy when doctors wondered whether his disease might be communicable. He not only ignored doctors' counsel to abstain from sex but after sex he even showed partners his lesions: "'Gay cancer,' he said, almost as if talking to himself. 'I've got gay cancer,' he'd say. 'I'm going to die and so are you.'"[12]

That he had been epidemiologically linked to 40 of the first 248 men identified with what was then called "Gay-Related Infectious Disease" (GRID) and that he ignored counsels to refrain from sexual relations made Dugas a prime target for explanations requiring a villain behind the epidemic. And acceptance of the characterization of Dugas as a villain has carried over even to accounts otherwise critical of Shilts's work. English professor James Miller, for example, observes, "I still shudder— whether with voyeuristic pleasure or zero-at-the-bone fright I can't tell—whenever I recall the lurid bathhouse scene where Patient Zero exchanges bodily fluids with a Castro Street clone and then cackles vampirically as he reveals his fulminant lesions: 'I've got gay cancer. . . . I'm going to die and so are you.'"[13] In describing Dugas's behavior in bathhouses, however, Shilts uses adverbs and adjectives sparingly. Only in describing Dugas's sexual willfulness does Shilts freely avail himself of a more expansive characterization, offering motives and attitudes.[14] Thus the spare description of the bathhouse scenes permits and elicits varying reactions. Though some readers have found Dugas a vengeful, viral sadist, it is not clear whether Dugas's remark that his partner is going to die means that Dugas has successfully caused disease in this partner or whether, in the fullness of sexual time, the partner cannot hope to avoid the disease because gay life is the way it is, because the partner already has the disease, or because the disease is unavoidable in any case.[15] Certainly, Shilts does not have Dugas cackling; on the contrary, he is talking almost to himself, whatever that might mean to a partner dressing hastily at his side, whatever that partner might have known—if anything—about gay cancer and its meaning for his own fate.

Despite the caution Shilts exhibits about directly attributing malevolent motives to Dugas in bathhouse scenes, he nevertheless stacks the narrative cards against Dugas from the beginning. There is little in Shilts's presentation that might exculpate Dugas or mitigate the view that Dugas, either in his person or in the ideals he epitomized, bore significant

responsibility for the epidemic. It even appears that Shilts has characterized Dugas as the Aristotelian efficient cause of the epidemic, insofar
as he appears as its mechanism of transmission in this country, and gay
ideals were the formal cause of the epidemic insofar as they shaped the
culture in which transmission could occur easily. Shilts directs the reader's
blame toward Dugas when he reports that one physician investigated
legal measures to prevent Dugas from having sex and that strangers
accosted Dugas on the street and told him to leave town. The narrative,
moreover, cues the reader to identify with Dugas's "innocent" sexual
partner. At one point, for example, Shilts describes Dugas's behavior in
a bathhouse this way: "He would have sex with *you,* turn up the lights
in the cubicle, and point out his Kaposi's sarcoma lesions."[16] By breaking
the third-person narrative form here—the form typical of journalistic
reporting—Shilts invites the reader to imagine being Dugas's victim.
Such an invitation would be more readily accepted, of course, by readers
prepared to imagine themselves open to gay sex and to bathhouses. Such
an invitation may work in other readers to elicit a homophobic overlay
to whatever other moral hostility they may feel about Dugas's behavior.
The scenes even invite a conflation of homosexuality with promiscuity
with callous, endangering behavior. This identification is amplified in its
evocative force since Shilts never once cues the reader to empathize with
whatever doubt and suffering Dugas must have endured during his
sickness. Even Dugas's incredulity about the communicability of his
condition—who had ever known cancer could be contagious?—is cast
as denial; precious little sympathy is given to the skepticism Dugas might
have had about the communicability of a hitherto unknown pathologic
syndrome.[17] The social prestige and moral authority of medicine are
powerful forces to be sure, but even so it would be hard to believe that
medicine could produce new categories of disease. Shilts did not in fact
interview Dugas (if such an interview was possible before Dugas's death),
and there is no sympathetic word uttered by anyone on his behalf in the
entire massive volume. In fact, Shilts does not offer Dugas as a portrait
in biography so much as a one-dimensional scoundrel in a gothic novel,
an occasion for lamentation about the evils of (gay) men.

Dugas's individual failings are not Shilts's only targets of criticism.
Despite the claim that he is merely reporting, Shilts clearly fictionalizes
Dugas's life as an emblem and symbol for gay life and especially for
excesses imputed to it. If Dugas is blameworthy in the origins of the
epidemic, by extension so too is the sexual ethos of gay life itself, because
Shilts uses Dugas, and especially his willful sexuality, as a figure for all

gay men. Shilts says, for example, that Dugas had achieved what *every* man wanted from gay life. In his liberated life-style Dugas had freedom, travel, drugs, and plenty of sex. He was therefore the incarnation of gay male desire; only accidents of circumstance block other gay men from living like, desiring like, and being desired like Dugas. According to such a characterization, Dugas represented and gay culture pursued as its ideal that promiscuous, emotionally and materially unencumbered hedonism that opened the door to the epidemic. Fleshy immersion in sexuality was not merely accidental to Dugas's nature. Shilts says: "Sex wasn't just sex to Gaetan; sex was who Gaetan was—it was the basis of his identity."[18] To the extent then that Shilts uses Dugas as a figure for gay men—no other gay man in *And the Band Played On* is said to represent what every man wanted from gay life; not an activist, not a politician, not a journalist—the very defining properties of gay life provide the conditions of the epidemic's possibility. In an ideal gay world it would only be a matter of time before everyone slept with everyone—"so many men, so little time," lamented the motto of the age—with the result that there was nothing in gay sexual identity or its pursuits that would be a natural obstacle to or conscriptable ally against the epidemic.

According to this psychofictional characterization of gay life in *And the Band Played On*, gay males were not only vulnerable to the epidemic because of the ways in which they shared their bodies but also because they would be individually (like Dugas) and collectively (like bathhouse owners) compelled to resist measures to control the epidemic because of the way in which gay identity had been so narrowly defined and constructed. Control of the epidemic thus meant an undermining of gay identity by asking gay men to give up the sexual habits that had given them self-identification, self-affirmation, escape from oppressive personal histories, and the possibility of new forms of community.[19] By this logic any counsel or legal mandate to refrain from sex would have to be opposed by gay men as an assault on the foundations of individual and collective gay identity. It would follow that gay men would find counsel against gay sex, even if intended to protect their health, fulsomely resonant with echoes of moralistic and medical judgments that condemned gay sex as immoral, illegal, and even mentally disordered. So if the *very nature* of gay identity proved an obstacle to its own protection from the epidemic, then the conceptual foundations are laid for the protection of gay men from themselves by others, by public health authorities, for example, who would have to disregard gay protest. And indeed Shilts plots the bathhouse controversy in his analysis exactly along these lines.

Shilts concludes his "description" of Dugas, saying: "In any event, there's no doubt that Gaetan played a key role in spreading the new virus from one end of the United States to the other. The bathhouse controversy, peaking so dramatically in San Francisco on the morning of his death, was also linked to Gaetan's own exploits in those sex palaces and his recalcitrance in changing his ways."[20] Shilts sees Dugas here less as a person than as a kind of sexual constellation whose points of infection across the nation had been connected by the departure and arrival schedules of airline timetables. Certainly, Shilts sees Dugas as having achieved what every man desired from gay life, but at his death, Shilts says, "he had become what every man feared."[21] Dugas no longer belonged to gay culture in particular as its ideal but instead belonged to the world as a universal human threat, joining an elite rank of global terrors alongside nuclear destruction, biochemical warfare, and ecological calamity, every one of them linked with the specter of mass death.

Is Dugas what every man need fear? Even if one adopts a purely journalistic stance in regard to the life of Gaetan Dugas, there are other ways in which the story might have been told. Dugas was, after all, but a flight attendant without any particular history of moral strength; he lived unascetically in a culture that does not require sexual self-mortification. Claims about the transmissibility of cancer and of a new, previously unknown immune disorder would have been hard to believe even among those inclined to sexual asceticism. And even if Dugas had acknowledged his condition, in advance, to his sexual partners, it is unclear whether there would have been any more or any fewer cases of AIDS in the United States. Shilts offers no evidence that Dugas was specifically responsible for a diagnosis of AIDS in another person after being advised to refrain from sex. He does not cite a case of AIDS that would not have occurred otherwise except for the sinister bathhouse malevolence of that Canadian flight attendant betraying the obligatory altruism of his profession. In some respects too it was purely accidental that Gaetan Dugas became "Patient Zero." There were (and are) other gay men whose lives and exploits replicated his, whose address books held as many if not more names and telephone numbers, who were addicted in the etymological sense of the word (addicted meaning "assenting") to bathhouses, whose looks and sexuality were equally a career unto themselves. In many ways Dugas lived no differently from many of the continent-hopping, urban peers of his time. Why therefore should the hammer of judgment fall as heavily on Dugas as Shilts's narrative requires, especially since such a judgment replicates the homophobia that equates homoeroticism with AIDS, especially since a large measure of Dugas's "fault" was not that he lived differently from others but merely that he—not they—got "it" first?

The claim that links Dugas to the emergence of AIDS in the United States is worth considering critically. Shilts reports that "at least 40 of the first 248 gay men diagnosed with GRID in the United States, as of April 12, 1982, either had sex with Gaetan Dugas or had sex with someone who did."[22] He further remarks that "a [Centers for Disease Control (CDC)] statistician calculated the odds on whether it could be coincidental that 40 of the first 248 gay men to get GRID might all have had sex either with the same man or with men sexually linked to him. The statistician figured that the chance did not approach zero—it was zero."[23] We do not know how the statistician made his or her calculations, but at one point a mean incubation period for the disease—the time between infection and emergence of symptoms—is stipulated as 10.5 months.[24] Such an assumption might support the claim that Dugas's role in infection in others could not be coincidental, but the measurement of latency in this way is meaningless since Shilts himself reports that infections could in fact date to 1976 (four years prior to Dugas's diagnosis), in which case the attributions of AIDS to sex with Dugas cannot be proved. A long latency period would in fact increase the likelihood of coincidence and diminish the certainty of causal connection. Certainly, the case for Dugas's causal role in the epidemic is far less convincing than Shilts represents it.

Dugas was certainly not exemplary in his behavior, but it is hard to say that his weaknesses were especially glaring given the times, given the nature and nurture of homoerotic desire in the United States. And whatever moral weaknesses he may have had were certainly amplified by the contrivances of contemporary culture. Easy airline flights across oceans and continents, for example, have had as much to do with the communicability of AIDS as much as any other epidemiological vector, including erotic ones. Perhaps the interesting question to ask about Dugas is not how one man continued to engage in risky behavior even after learning of his dangerous, communicable condition but why this story made its way into media reports and histories of the epidemic rather than reports on the deaths of gay men and analyses of the oppressive conditions of culture that contributed in a prejudicial way to the forms of gay identity in the United States which made gay men susceptible to infection. Why is it so easy to believe that the villainy of a few persons (or a class of persons) caused an epidemic through their deliberate behavior? Why is it that social contributions to the epidemic (in the form of increasing opportunities for sexual interaction) and medical contributions (in the form of increased control of other sexually communicable diseases) are ignored as relevant in assessing the "causes" of the epidemic? Focusing on Gaetan Dugas and his "personal" responsibility serves only to mystify the many forces that are the context, the unacknowledged preconditions, and sometimes the unknowable impetus of all human choices. Moreover, the synecdochic use of Dugas for gay men in general clearly risks making an anti-AIDS campaign into an antigay campaign.

There are, of course, people diagnosed with HIV infection or AIDS who do share beds and needles with unwarned others. But to focus on specific persons—individually or as a group—as responsible for the epidemic structures the analysis so as to avoid identifying other important preconditions of HIV infection. While condemnation of people who "spread AIDS," for example, is common, discussion about people who "contract" HIV by reason of failure to protect themselves is infinitely less common. Certain social responses show that even among people with HIV, blame is assigned in morally revealing ways. The ovations confirming Earvin "Magic" Johnson's standing as a national hero following the announcement of his HIV infection, for example, suggest that if there is villainy to be assigned in the epidemic, it does not very often go to the people who are "innocently" on the receiving end of an infection. The very terminology of "spreading" AIDS—terminology that is ubiquitously, unconsciously prevalent—suggests the premeditated, active transmission of disease to passive, innocent victims. The asymmetry revealed in the prevalence of language about "spreading" HIV and the comparative dearth of language about "contracting" the infection suggests that a cultural assumption is at work which believes that but for a malevolent few individuals—like Dugas—there would be no further "spread" of HIV. Such a presumption, however, is not only untrue to the facts of human nature, because it fails to acknowledge the way in which all persons are susceptible to some degree of erotic risks of infection, but also works as an obstacle for HIV education by imposing the responsibility for "containment" of the epidemic on a few persons whose duty it is to remain isolated in their viral quarantine. This kind of moral expectation—that people with HIV bear the burden of protecting all others—strategically relieves all others of duties in their own behalf, and the world is thus made safe once again for the noninfected and made safe in a way that requires no effort from the uninfected other than their contribution to the conceptual design of a moral quarantine.

We might also ask why Gaetan Dugas is represented as a greater social evil than, say, educational failures that even today leave teenagers confused about and unskilled in effective ways of protecting themselves against HIV infection. Some people (including prostitutes) with HIV infection have in fact been jailed here and there around the country when they have been found to have had sexual relations with others, and bathhouses have been closed in some cities. But what is the import of these events? That "johns" and bathhouse patrons have a *right* to sex without risks of HIV? That the *duty* of the public is to be outraged at sex and needle use among people with HIV? That public authority should be omnipresent to guarantee that all sex and needle use is without risk of HIV infection?

Narratives about individuals who "spread" AIDS offer easily identifiable culprits on whom to pin the blame for the epidemic and its continuing calamities. Shilts does make clear in his narrative that there is plenty of blame to go around for the epidemic—and he certainly does not spare some gay activists in this regard—but his depiction of Dugas's involvement with its beginnings is too facile. Shilts does not show, for example, the way in which human lives are socially intertwined and the extent to which human "choices" or identities are artifacts of culture. He does not read Dugas against the background of human fallibility, that fallibility that has sunk the best of both persons and nations, their best intentions notwithstanding. He does not read the sexual "fast lane" against the difficult emergence of gay culture in Western history.[25] Instead, the life of Gaetan Dugas is "reported" as a kind of sexual vortex whirling in a moral solipsism indifferent to the health and lives of others. Dugas hovers as a menacing, inverted incubus over the sleepy, dreamy sex play of gay men. To the extent that such a picture emerges and to the extent that Dugas serves as a figure for all gay men in this narrative, responsibility for the epidemic not unsurprisingly falls to individuals rather than to culture at large. Such a depiction also suggests that the reform or control of certain persons and places would restore what is otherwise a planet and a civilization in preordained moral and immunological equilibrium.

AIDS and the Body Politic

The conceptualization of the origins of the epidemic is instructive in the way in which blame is fixed and the catastrophe understood. If AIDS is thought to follow the collapse of will—in either individuals or in the class of gay men and drug-users as a whole—such a view invites speculation about the necessity of controls that would restrict the range of sexual and civic choices traditionally respected in moral and political philosophy. Monroe Price's *Shattered Mirrors,* for example, fleshes out this kind of speculation, foretelling what the epidemic might mean for the future understanding of citizenship, rights, and freedom. Put at risk by AIDS, he says, are the equation between autonomy and sexual expression; the accustomed, limited role of government authority in shaping public thinking and morality; the fragile standing of minorities in American society; and the circumspect and rational use of government power. Given such a view, the continued elusiveness of either cure or vaccine may yet further wither faith in the state and its ideals; in desperation, public opinion may swing in favor of more drastic measures of control.[26] Price's book is full of proleptic prophecy that fear of the epidemic, limited success in containing the "spread" of AIDS, the traditional wide berth given to government action justified in the name of public well-being, and a brooding public opinion all threaten to provoke an assault on civil liberties as well as reconfigure an understanding of the meaning of American civic traditions.

Ronald Bayer has also advanced the view that AIDS may prove a pivot on which the nation could turn against its commitment to reason and civic traditions: Will reason, balance, and a search for modest but effective intervention, he wonders, fall victim to a rancorous din?[27] Thus we can understand the gloss he puts on a California referendum that would have put restrictions on the employment of people with HIV infections. Although the bill was in fact defeated, Bayer says, the referendum "revealed how popular discontent might be exploited in the years ahead as the absolute numbers of AIDS cases mounted. It had also demonstrated the existence of a popular base that could be mobilized for a repressive turn in public policy."[28] The conclusion of Bayer's *Private Acts, Social Consequences* also raises the question of whether the American public will at some time demand tougher, less voluntary measures against AIDS; it also points out the ease with which a voluntarist strategy for prevention of infection might be subverted.[29]

In one sense these kinds of analyses are merely tautologies that AIDS cannot but change the future. Time and again they fall back on the language of "may," "could," "can," and "might" and thus trade in the realm of logical possibilities. Fear of the endangerment of the nation "by" AIDS can, as Price says, muffle concern about constitutional formalities and the protection of rights, but such a claim would be true about *any* durable and deep fear held in the nation, whether about AIDS or oil supplies.[30] It is *always* true that society might suffer mood swings in which it is prepared to jettison its carefully crafted legal precedents, its civic traditions, and the roles it expects of government, and this is no less true in and because of the AIDS epidemic. Yet society might respond otherwise to AIDS. Society might come to accept the burdens of AIDS as part of the human condition and not see the disease as requiring a special moral interpretation or the imposition of coercive measures. The epidemic might elicit untapped reserves of social altruism rather than transmogrify society into a punitive if "enlightened" garrison. Gay philosopher Richard D. Mohr has suggested that "ideas, thoughts, reason, and argument will have no significant role to play either in the formation of public policy or in changing individual behavior in the AIDS crisis."[31] His view of the future suggests that profoundly antigay values and structures in society will work to confound an honest confrontation of the epidemic. In this foretelling, a future beset by AIDS becomes not an aberration of contemporary society but its logical conclusion. At their worst, analyses, which raise dark visions of the future but do not equivalently argue against the evils of such a future, risk being self-fulfilling prophecies by reason of the very fears they create and popularize.

Looming behind many analyses of the influence of AIDS on the future is the sense that the real damages of the epidemic have yet to transpire. These analyses are often cast in terms of protecting the future from the present epidemic, as if the evils of the epidemic belonged most significantly, perhaps even exclusively, to the future. For example, one of the most alarmist analyses of AIDS is to be found in Gene Antonio's *The AIDS Cover-Up?*[32] which was published during a 1986 peak in national AIDS anxiety. Antonio argued that AIDS is more dangerous than plague or a major war because of the silent way in which it "spreads." In what he called "optimistic" projections, based on his own calculations, Antonio estimated that by the end of 1990 there would be sixty-four million infected Americans in addition to mass death, mass sickness, and a crushed and wasted health system.[33] Along the same lines, Finnish philosophers Heta Häyry and Matti Häyry called for action against AIDS in the name of the millions of people in the future who may fall victim to it. To make their point, they aver that "nuclear holocaust, the main source of fear among people today, will tomorrow look like the only peaceful way out of our misery if governments do not care to stop the triumphant march of AIDS *now*."[34] What dangers AIDS must pose if nuclear holocaust could in any way ever be a consolation! But if the dangers of the epidemic do belong primarily to the future, is not the political and moral effect to dismiss the urgency of AIDS? Rhetoric of this kind and pitch—ranged alongside the hyperbole typical in political analyses competing with all other world events for attention—could suggest that AIDS is not yet sufficiently important to require systematic concern, that it has not yet killed enough persons to justify trimming the budgets of other, important government expenses. Viewing the epidemic as a future harm not only provokes exaggerated depictions of its gravity but it also and ironically drains off energy and resources by situating the epidemic in some remote period distant from the interests and concerns of *present* life. Certainly, depicting nuclear holocaust as a "solution" preferable to a future with AIDS risks writing AIDS into the order of fate as a cataclysm against which no human effort could prevail regardless of how much money government set aside for AIDS-prevention programs. Situating the epidemic primarily in the future permits both an exaggeration and trivialization of the epidemic and in either case risks muting the current significance of AIDS.

Conjoined with a view of the future despoiled by the misuse of civil liberties meant for pursuits far nobler than bathhouse sex and drug use, it is little surprising that there would be analyses like those of Price and Bayer regarding the possibility of extensive civic revisionism which would brusquely assert public control over individual choice. Price observes that "law becomes a gracious song that can be sung when it is possible to sing but abandoned when it is not."[35] If people with HIV continue to threaten society with their disease, the subtext of this message reads, society must revert to an atavistic standard somehow morally superior to the excesses of contemporary civic traditions that are special and apparently temporary dispensations from a more compelling moral authority whose name is the public health or common weal. A concomitant consequence of depictions of "future AIDS" is that the moral and social intensity they would ostensibly marshall may be defused by the oracular futurity of their messages.

A "Scientific" Future

Discussions about the future of AIDS do not belong, of course, only to historians and political moralists. They are also to be found in science and the media. Reports from the 1992 international AIDS conference, held in Amsterdam,[36] raised the future of AIDS in ways that not only replayed earlier forms of AIDS discussion but that also situated the import of the epidemic in the future.

Researchers at that conference held out little hope for an immediate cure or a vaccine,[37] and they forecast a disheartening AIDS toll. Since many predictions were prepared for the year 2000 the feared future of AIDS draws nearer all the time. An article in *U.S. News & World Report*, for example, said: "Researchers at the Harvard AIDS Institute expect that by the year 2000, the number of Thais afflicted with HIV will balloon to 2 to 4 million out of a current population of 58 million, largely through heterosexual intercourse."[38] The same piece said of AIDS in India: "Despite official statistics that calculate just 125 victims, an un-counted 6,000 people are now believed to be dying of AIDS in the country, with another 500,000 to 1 million people infected with HIV."[39] Worldwide estimates for the year 2000 were put at between 30 and 110 million people with HIV infection by 2000. By now, of course, ever-worsening prognostications are standard features of narratives about AIDS in almost all disciplines. The costs of treating people with AIDS also form part of the archetype of AIDS forecasting.[40] The future of the world's economy is often called into question as well: "The pernicious plague, now spreading misery around the world at an alarm-ing rate, may also plunder the global economy over the next decade."[41] Litanies about the evils of AIDS offered by political commentators, religious leaders, and writers to Dear Abby invariably include AIDS among the woes of our age which imperil the future.

Beyond these fairly typical features of AIDS discussions, reports from the Amsterdam conference also raised the specter of a third virus re-sponsible for patients with apparent AIDS who failed to demonstrate evidence of HIV infection. Several AIDS researchers reported the ex-istence of such patients,[42] and one researcher said that he had even isolated a new virus from the patients.[43] Other researchers withheld comment about their findings pending the publication of reports in scientific journals.[44] The possibility of a novel pathogen fueled even further speculation about the future of worldwide AIDS. First, such reports called into question the state of biomedical knowledge about the pathogenesis of AIDS; they raised questions about the aggressiveness of the CDC in monitoring information and trends in this epidemic and about the worth of embargoes against release of research data to the media prior to publication in biomedical journals. Mostly, though, these reports questioned whether current measures taken to protect blood products can be effective against an unidentified pathogen. Even the earliest reports about a possible third pathogen responsible for AIDS took pains to stave off panic about an "uncontrolled" epidemic. Several researchers pointed out, for example, that the new cases of "AIDS" may prove to be other forms of unrecognized immune disorders, the product of an increased vigilance for such disorders. Others pointed out that blood banks should be protected by virtue of the steps they already take to avoid pathogen-bearing blood. A *New York Times* lead editorial cautioned against panic at the identification of a new "AIDS virus." The thirty-some cases of idiopathic AIDS, the *Times* concluded, are not yet a threat and may never be: "The strange new AIDS-like cases may yet turn out to be more a scientific curiosity than a public health hazard."[45]

Contradictory reports about the contagiousness of AIDS viruses, however many of them there may be, also appeared in 1992. *Newsweek,* for example, said: "If there *is* a new AIDS virus, it doesn't appear any more contagious than HIV. Some of the stricken patients may deny having HIV risk factors, but there's no evidence that they have contracted, or transmitted, their illness through casual contact."[46] A report of HIV in Thailand, however, suggested that there were HIV "subtypes" that differed not only in "virulence" but also in contagiousness.[47]

The combined effect of all these reports is striking inasmuch as they underscore the role of authority and science in predicting AIDS ills and deepening the mystery over the disease without being able to offer any substantive biomedical control over the current and future epidemic. Against a predicted, global catastrophe of proportions not yet imaginable, the reports of novel occurrences of AIDS outside the reigning explanatory paradigm threaten a revolution against the confident authority of AIDS expertise. It is as if medicine owes as much to Cassandra as to Asklepios. Hence the rush to calm the public is accompanied by reports of a new virus that might elude the barriers ensuring the safety of blood used in transfusions and other medical applications. Uncertainty invites speculation, and where there is speculation people will see in the future what salvific qualities they think necessary for the redemption of the present as well as what catastrophes they think inevitable from current, objectionable practices. Certainly it is true that there have been many false leads regarding the pathogenesis of AIDS, and there are many reasons not to rush to judgment about the significance of cases of idiopathic AIDS and about questions of subtype virulence and transmissibility. Nonetheless, that the future remains the pervasive worry about AIDS suggests the many ways in which AIDS is not felt in the present, the many ways in which the epidemic is undervalued as the evil that it is at present. It is certainly telling that in all the major media reports about a possible new pathogen, no one thought to mention the significance of that conjecture for people who suffered from that kind of disorder. Amid all the speculations about future victims of this virus, there was no mention of those who might already be affected.[48] Medicine and moral civilization apparently have no interest in such PWAs or their loss is already without significance. They are already apparently beyond the pale in a sense consonant with the origins of that phrase: pale, from the Latin word for stake and thus fence, in a phrase originally referring to the limits of the English empire in Ireland; a boundary beyond which civilization has no interest.

Conceptualizing the relationship between AIDS and the future is a problematic task. Certainly there is much to be done to protect future generations from the ravages of the epidemic. Yet invocation of the future may in fact serve other strategies that work against such protection, strategies that distance the epidemic from its immediacy, strategies whose hyperbole corrodes commitment to or even belief in the possibility of overcoming the epidemic, and strategies that in sum write off the present as beyond redemption. Such strategies may also "read" the epidemic into nature, suggesting that it is the order of nature, not the social order, that stretches the epidemic over the globe and concluding that human efforts of resistance are as of little use as trying to halt continental drift. We must even consider motives for the protection of the future: Is "public health" merely the continuation of politics by other means? Does "the future" have the same kind of coded meaning as "family values" and imply specific moral arrangements of human relations and only those?

The future, of course, has not been imagined only as an immunological dystopia in the style of, for example, German novelist Peter Zingler's *Die Seuche* (The Plague), in which a future society is highly polarized by HIV and Germany's extremist "solutions" to the epidemic.[49] On the contrary, there have been works of imagination which have tried to foresee a future protected from AIDS without at the same time invoking specters of mass death, of foretelling a world laid waste by bodily fluids. Often focusing on the political activism of people with AIDS, gay men, and their allies,[50] these works try to imagine a future *without* AIDS which links past and future in community with the present. One such act of imagination may be found in the final moments of the

1990 movie *Longtime Companion,* by Craig Lucas and Norman René. In that scene two lovers, Willy and Fuzzy, walk the beach with Fuzzy's sister and discuss demonstrations, arrests, their losses, and their conceits. "I just wanna be there if they ever do find a cure," Willy tells his companions. "Can you imagine what it would be like?" Fuzzy wonders. A pregnant moment later a swarm of the "dead" rushes over the hill toward the trio, full of sound, color, and life. James Miller has observed that in such an ending "all losses are restored and sorrows end in an extemporaneous party scene that recaptures the joie de vivre of the Fire Island revelers at the beginning of the film, minus, of course, the poppers and booze and virus."[51] As an act of imagination and as one of the very few, sustained cinematic features about AIDS, *Longtime Companion* could not be expected to fulfill all hopes, and the movie faced criticism not only for its rich, white character demographics but also for the escapism of its all-too-utopian ending.[52] *Longtime Companion* does not offer a future ravaged medically and politically by AIDS. Neither, though, does it offer merely an escapist, apolitical revery, merely an AZT-laced opiate for the masses. The future envisioned by these long-time companions is no religiously earned "compensation" for present trials and sufferings, no delayed gratification deserved through virtuous living. Instead, the ending of *Longtime Companion* enacts a momentary dissolution of time and thereby robs it of any capacity to frame invidious conflicts between the past, present, and future. Judgments about the origin of AIDS disappear as insignificant because some future cure has for a moment reached into the past. The protection of the future cannot serve as a pretext for any political cause since there is no other moment but this one. Questions about blame for the past and responsibility for the future also collapse in this scene because—except that these terms are no longer meaningful—the "living" embrace the "dead" in a temporally indivisible community.

An observation by the seventeenth-century French philosopher Blaise Pascal may have an uncanny relevance to this postmodern epidemic. In the *Pensées* Pascal commented on the human condition: "We almost never think of the present, and if we do think of it, it is only to see what light it throws on our plans for the future. The present is never our end. The past and present are our means, the future alone our end." In our studied avoidance of the present, Pascal observed, we (whom he called "thinking reeds") fill our lives with vanities and diversions: "Thus we never actually live, but hope to live."[53] Controlling our penchant to see our lives through lenses of the past and future can itself determine whether we live or only and merely *hope to live* in and with the epidemic. There are many ways in which to tell the story of the origin of AIDS, and there are many ways to imagine its future. But there is certainly a lethal combination in the view that people with HIV are themselves alone morally responsible for the "spread" of the epidemic and in the view that the "real" dangers of the epidemic have yet to transpire. Against such narratives, we would be wise to underscore human fallibility in determining responsibility for the emergence of this divisive epidemic. It would certainly be unwise and unfair to hold out a future so damaged by AIDS as to indulge rightist fantasies of stern "anti-AIDS" measures or to characterize the evils of the epidemic as not yet having "really" happened. Shilt's depiction of Gaetan Dugas may satisfy the anthropo-morphizing desire for an explanation of evil, and the lure of "get tough" politics may satisfy the hunger for assurance that "something" will be done to protect the immunological and economic purity of the future, but narratives emphasizing "individual responsibility" and "future dam-age" prevent seeing the many complex social forces that to this day conspire to permit further HIV infection as well as ways in which the epidemic has yet—future damage apart—to be appreciated as the dam-age it already, irrevocably is. In this epidemic imagined another way, time does not have to be viewed as either the engine of willful conspiracy or the horizon of inevitable tragedy. In an epidemic thus understood as something other than an antagonism between the past and the future, hope may proceed in the name of a people undivided by time.

2

The Search for a Cure

The search for a cure for AIDS has raised important ethical questions about access to drugs and experimentation with new medication. Some PWA organizations, for example, demand full access to all drugs that show any therapeutic benefit; others have even rejected the distinction between experiment and therapy altogether.[1] One of the founding motives of ACT UP, according to its founder, gay writer Larry Kramer, was to get drugs into the bodies of PWAs.[2] While treatment by orthodox medicine has vastly improved since the beginning of the epidemic, in 1994 biomedicine still cannot offer predictable control over AIDS, much less any therapy that amounts to a decisive cure. Given the desperation of PWAs for a cure, it is not surprising that quackery has found a thriving business. PWAs have sought relief in diverse and unlikely nutritional regimens, exercise programs, blood-heating techniques, faith healing, and assorted psychodynamic approaches. They have sought cures wherever there is hope for sale. By contrast, some policy analysts have called for more stringent control over access to drugs and more reliance on the "gold standard" of double-blind trials, which include control groups receiving no drug, only a placebo, as a means of demonstrating the actual efficacy of drugs under experimental review.[3] Critics of an open-access drug policy decry as futile any pharmaceutical research and treatment carried out on an ad hoc basis, and they insist on the importance of painstaking standards of biomedical research as the only pathway toward progress, even if that progress amounts merely to consumer protection from useless and dangerous "remedies," even if that progress cannot promise to secure the life of anyone now living with AIDS.

Narratives by and about PWAs are less sanguine about the process and progress of orthodox medicine. In these accounts the search for a treatment is always obstinate, often quixotic, sometimes dangerous, and ultimately futile, as the narratives to be discussed here make abundantly clear. Conflict between PWAs (trying to keep themselves individually healthy) and bench scientists (trying to identify treatments effective on randomly selected groups) is likely to continue as long as no wholly efficacious treatments for HIV-related conditions emerge. But besides the troubling ethical concern about access to experimental therapies and the design of clinical trials, there is another important ethical concern: the effect of the search for a cure for AIDS on PWAs and on gay PWAs in particular. Thus far the search for an AIDS cure has not only proved an ambiguous benefit to PWAs, it has sometimes even brought cognizable harm. I do not wish say that both orthodox and alternative medicine have not brought relief and solace to many PWAs, for they undeniably have, but the relentless search for treatment and a cure does sometimes open PWAs to new vistas of suffering and hopelessness they would not otherwise know. Hope may also be an iatrogenic suffering.

Borrowing Time

On the very first page of his 1988 *Borrowed Time* Paul Monette says, "I take my drug from Tijuana twice a day."[4] This unspecified drug came from Mexico because, no doubt, it had not been approved for use in the United States or was substantially cheaper there. Either way, this admission is an affront to medical and pharmaceutical practices in this country which force PWAs to rely on the sometimes illegal drugs of a developing nation in order to secure their health. The depiction of medicine in the rest of Monette's memoir of a lover and friends looking for a cure only deepens that challenge. Consciously and unconsciously, the memoir documents how the search for an AIDS cure opens PWAs and their lovers and advocates to unreasoning hope and subjects them to the depredations of institutional medicine and what homophobia abides there.

While Monette and his lover, Roger Horwitz, do encounter some caring and compassionate individuals in their search for treatment, Monette more typically represents the institutions and practitioners of medicine as consistently failing them across the range of their needs as gay men worried about, sick with, and dying with AIDS. Inasmuch as the memoir amounts to a virtual catalog of the damages of medicine, those few patches of text offered on behalf of the humanity and accomplishment of medicine are rare oases indeed. More often, Monette scores traditional medicine, especially the operations of its experimental arm. At the beginning of Roger's illness, for example, medical uncertainty about the nature and significance of AIDS permitted patients some hope that would eventually prove ill founded. While talk about the fatality of AIDS was in the air, its symptoms were so unclear that gay men did not understand what medical problems qualified for diagnosis as AIDS proper. Monette cannot understand, for example, how his friend Cesar Albini's swollen, unhealing leg is related to the rare pneumonia and cancer that were the conditions first gropingly identified as AIDS.[5] Similarly, Roger's minor cough and a not-very-serious swelling in Paul's neck lead them worriedly to physicians, who told them that their symptoms did not match the criteria set forth for AIDS, that they did not even qualify for something called at the time pre-AIDS. Such epistemological uncertainty about the nature of the syndrome on the one hand functioned to make gay men worry unrelievedly about whether they had the fatal illness while on the other hand offered them false hope when practitioners could not identify their illnesses as AIDS-related. While it would be unfair to blame medicine for its uncertainty about a newly emerging viral syndrome, the effect of that uncertainty was to create informational and educational vacuums in the public at large and to permit diagnostic imprecision in the clinic as well as false hopes in its clients. Uncertainty about the nature of AIDS and the uncertain distinction between pre-AIDS and AIDS itself comes to a farcical collapse in *Borrowed Time* when one of Monette's friends dies with doctors all around insisting that while they did not know exactly what it was that killed him, it certainly was not AIDS.[6] How many more, Monette wonders, died but never made the lists?[7] In an even more ironic twist, one of the very physicians whose reports signaled the formal 1981 beginning of the U.S. epidemic wrongly told Monette his symptoms would probably prove to be nothing.[8]

The HIV-related sickness and death of Cesar Albini and Roger Horwitz are shadowed with iatrogenic suffering. Roger undergoes many of the predictable blood tests, X-rays, CAT scans, invasive and disabling bronchoscopies, and takes home the grocery bags of drugs that are the medical fate of PWAs, all of which inflict burdens of one kind or another on him; at one point both Roger and Paul are misdiagnosed with amoebiasis. Monette criticizes the depersonalization that occurs in hospital settings: the stripping away of personal identity, the reduction of the individual to a medical problem. Many of the health-care difficulties experienced by Monette and Roger are not, of course, limited to PWAs. Physicians elsewhere make mistakes, misdiagnose patients, and cannot promise to cure all human ills. Not only can physicians not treat all conditions, they often fail to approach individual patients in sympathetic ways. New interns do all appear improbably young and interchangeable, and they often relate to patients only through newly learned questions that crudely impose a biomedical framework on the unscientifically ordered lives of their patients; encounters between sick men and women who construct stories of their sickness in relation to their personal biographies often clash in narrative entanglements with physicians who try to see diseases and disorders apart from those personal histories. Many people cannot afford the luxuries of private medical care and must seek recourse in the limited health-care services available at publicly supported hospitals.

But AIDS produces its own unique circumstances in this account too. After Roger is hospitalized, he undergoes a bronchoscopy, in which a tube is inserted through the throat into the lungs in order to retrieve a tissue sample for study. The experience is exceptionally painful but necessary in order to confirm certain diagnoses; the discomfort of this sadistic parody of fellatio[9] leaves Roger mute and racked with pain. Shortly after his first hospitalization, a physician appears in Roger's room and announces that tests do confirm *Pneumocystis* pneumonia, but he says no more. As Monette says, "The intern had never once said the word."[10] *Pneumocystis* served as a cultural code for AIDS, a code that permitted discussion of AIDS without the need for direct use of the term, a code that reflected the need even in medicine to discuss AIDS in an indirect fashion because of its unsavory social connections with gay sex, drug use, and immorality. Uncertainty about the nature of AIDS had previously permitted Roger and Paul to hope Roger was not affected, his symptoms notwithstanding. The intern's silence about AIDS might be motivated by sympathy, a wish to spare Roger the burden of a diagnosis that was as much a scandal as a threat to his life. But from Roger and Monette's perspective, the physician's diagnostic evasion was merely paralepsis, confirming AIDS while pretending not to mention it. Such a reined-in diagnosis offered no important benefit to them. The doctor's reluctance to use the word AIDS recapitulated social inattention to AIDS and foretold a doomed outcome. The diagnosis in any case plunged Roger and Paul into the larger uncertainty of coping with an entirely untreatable condition.

The diagnosis does launch Paul and Roger on a crusade for a cure. They are favored by their economic standing and intellectual acumen, and they know as much. They know other gay men with AIDS who do not have access to any experimental drug protocols, including one man who waited hours to see a doctor in a public hospital all the while knowing that the doctors had no clue about how to help him.[11] But the lovers' privileges do not come without a price, especially as all these experimental efforts not only do not save Roger's life but also endanger him and tether him inextricably to physicians and hospitals. Throughout the memoir Monette chronicles the reticulated network of the AIDS underground, an informal cluster of friends and activists who keep watch for the newest drugs, especially antivirals, those that would attack the infection itself. As Monette put it: "The struggle for the drug gave us a great surge of purpose that colored everything. Any news about any drug could cut through my blackest despair."[12] Attention to this grapevine earned Roger placement in two drug trials. The first, for suramin, started in a Zurichlike clinic, all quiet and fastidiously clean. For the promise of the drug trial and the presence of a gay doctor in this sheltering clinic, Monette was grateful, but the gratitude was tempered by the secrecy he and Roger felt necessary about the diagnosis. Roger once even moved to another room in order to prevent contact with a patient who knew him. While the trial went forward in these favored circumstances, however, Monette worried all the while that if this drug failed, there would be no magic bullet.[13]

The drug did fail both Roger and others around the country: "As for the suramin—water under the bridge which seemed more lethal with every report that came in. . . . I felt ridiculous and ashamed. I who had pushed suramin all summer as practically a miracle drug." But Monette decides his own connivance in getting Roger into this trial is forgivable since he was gullible while "others knew exactly what they were doing" in offering so toxic a drug.[14] Monette censures the way in which other test sites continued their suramin studies even after it was clear that the drug was too toxic: "There was even one doctor who kept his patients on suramin through the winter, even when we knew how lethal the side effects were, and even as the patients died off one by one."[15] In the end, even as the clinical drug trial offered the only hope then available in the armamentarium of orthodox medicine, such experimentation simultaneously underscored the vulnerability of PWAs and their lovers and advocates. Most important, it didn't help; it almost killed Roger.

But on the grapevine there was already word of another drug, something known as AL-721. A personal connection at UCLA—favoritism, really—got Roger into a study of that new drug, which proved to be AZT, and Monette turns to this trial with hope, undaunted by the first near-disaster: "The thrill of the undercover operation kept us going, and this at a time when AZT had the status of a Holy Grail in the AIDS underground."[16] Roger was apparently the first person west of the Mississippi to be treated with the drug; Monette calls him the AZT poster child. And like suramin before it, the drug held out hope where elsewhere there was none. For a time the drug appears to work; at least Roger's clinical condition improves. Soon an AZT culture starts to flourish everywhere, with the beepers of friends and strangers going off at four-hour intervals to remind people to take their medication. But the promise of the drug is not fulfilled, and Roger succumbs to various complaints: shingles, anxiety attacks, aphasia, dementia, and the increasing blindness that precedes his decline to death. But even that blindness was fought with an experimental surgery.[17]

Monette and Horwitz's search for treatments and a cure, problematic in any case by reason of the mysterious nature of AIDS, was complicated by their sexual identities too. Dated from the appearance of those *Morbidity and Mortality Weekly Reports* pointing out the unusual occurrence of *Pneumocystis* pneumonia and Kaposi's sarcoma in 1981, the AIDS epidemic formally began less than eight years after the contested decision by the American Psychiatric Association (APA) to remove homosexuality per se from its categories of mental disorders. Many gay men who came of age in the fifties, sixties, and the early seventies would not even have viewed that decision as their "liberation" (though some did) so much as a confirmation that sexual reorientation therapy was their own Tuskegee syphilis experiment, as evidence that medicine did not value them in their lives and loves and understood their worth only in relation to the outcome of medical experiments carried out on them, sometimes involuntarily. The search for a medical cure for homosexuality had led to some grotesque efforts in chemical and electrical aversive therapy, drug treatment, testicular transplants, and even brain surgery.[18] And the practice of conversion therapy has not disappeared even today.[19]

It is not surprising that when medical authorities announced the emergence of a new, pernicious syndrome attacking gay men, many would have received the news suspiciously, even skeptically. Was this new syndrome the next phase of medical homophobia? In the history of APA classification homosexuality was first claimed to be a sociopathic personality disorder, then a sexual disorder, then an ego-dystonia, and finally—as the vestigial form of this pathological classification—sexual-orientation distress. Was AIDS a continuation of the perceived biomedical agenda to link homoeroticism with pathology? And even if gay people did not have a specific skepticism about AIDS per se as a continuation of a pathologizing homophobia, still after sometimes hard rites of passage to adulthood they would nevertheless have difficulties returning to the care of social institutions knowing as they did that schools, churches, government, and even doctors often failed to acknowledge, protect, and nurture them.

While Monette does not report a physician or nurse refusing to treat a PWA because he or she was gay, we nonetheless recognize in *Borrowed Time* an expectation of homophobia from medical institutions and health-care workers. Monette mentions that in the past a gay man with any disease even faintly venereal would seek out a physician who was also "on the bus." In other words, he would seek out a gay physician in order to avoid embarrassment or in hope of some understanding, even what Monette punningly calls "fellow feeling."[20] Such an observation suggests the way in which gay men often do not believe that heterosexual physicians understand them or are prepared to tolerate the diseases that attend their sexual lives. Though medical professions may no longer profess the pathology of homoeroticism, many gay men still do not believe that they will be accepted in the kind of unconditional doctor-patient relationship afforded straight people. It was, after all, only in mid-1993—almost twenty-five years after the beginnings of gay liberation at Stonewall and twelve years after the announcement of the existence of AIDS—that the American Medical Association (AMA) voted to declare discrimination on the basis of sexual orientation unacceptable within that professional organization.[21] Even then, the policy statement met opposition. The entrenched homophobia of medicine is underlined in Monette's narrative by an anecdote about a physician who rolled his eyes in a way to make plain that Roger's father must have done something very wrong to have had not one but two gay sons, and with two different wives no less.[22] In such an adversarial context the question

"Are you a homosexual?"—even if asked by a conscientious doctor looking for a means of HIV infection—triggers every protective instinct in a gay man against a homophobic environment and can have the effect of alarming gay PWAs rather than convincing them that the question is posed in their best medical interest.

An openly gay doctor does appear at the UCLA medical center where Roger is being treated. Peter Wolf is one of the few health-care workers in this account who offers the two refuge from the fear of medical homophobia. In a number of instances the best care given to Roger comes from persons capable of imagining themselves or their relatives as PWAs, a perspective easy enough for someone gay or friendly with gay men. Of Peter Wolf Monette relates: "Explaining that he had been treating AIDS patients since his first day as a doctor, he spoke simply and feelingly of looking down at a stricken man in bed and thinking: 'This is me.'"[23] Later on, a nurse with a gay son exhibited a committed interest in the well-being of her PWAs "so maybe if someone ever has to take care of him, they'll treat him like a son."[24] There is also a kindly gay phlebotomist singled out by Monette for praise. By contrast, when Monette poured out his worries about Roger's diagnosis to his own straight physician and asked what to do, that doctor "shrugged his shoulders with a cavalier unconcern I can only attribute to his certainty that he was safe himself. I've seen that straight man's shrug a hundred times. 'Burn the sheets,'" he replied . . . and then added, "You live alone, you die alone."[25] Monette does not say that no straight doctor offered support and consideration—in this regard Monette has nothing but highest praise for Dennis Cope ("And not once in twenty months did he not have time"[26])—but by and large the institutions and practitioners of medicine in his account distanced themselves from PWAs. Medicine stands apart from PWAs in the way it functionally forces the burdens of learning about AIDS diagnoses and treatments onto PWAs themselves. It stands apart in the labored efforts of dentists to appear—against all evidence—comfortable in the infection-control procedures of mask, gloves, and warily executed contact. It stands apart in the promotion of therapeutic strategies that permit hope of the most dubious kind. In the expectation that increased visibility of gay health-care workers would lift some of this burden, the very first item of the "Founding Statement of People with AIDS/ARC" recommends that health professionals "who are gay come out, especially to their patients who have AIDS."[27] Their presence is expected to mitigate—as it does in fact in Monette's memoir—the homophobic context of medicine by diminishing the way in which the conventions of the closet compromise the care of gay people with AIDS.

Eventually, since this is a memoir and not a biography in progress, Roger's decline accelerates, with fevers and sweats, coughing, the collapse of injectable veins, a catheter implant for drug injection, the infection of the catheter, disorientation, and increasing need for nursing care and AIDS buddies. Nevertheless, Monette continued to believe in the miracle of AZT. It fell to Dr. Cope, Roger's doctor, to point out to Monette the significance of Roger's fourth bout with *Pneumocystis* pneumonia: "It wouldn't be the worst thing if this were the one that took him."[28] In his last conscious moments, Roger "speaks" to Paul one last time by fluttering his eyelids. Knowing that it is finally over, Paul goes home. Awakened later by the phone, he and Roger's mother listen to a nurse's voice speak through the electric gauze of the answering machine: Roger has died. The days of his experiments are over even as Paul's had scarcely begun.

The representations of medicine in *Borrowed Time* are, to be sure, colored by personal grief and anger, and medicine may be wrongly blamed for the evils that belong to human frailty more than personal iniquity, but these characterizations are instructive nevertheless about the meaning of the quest for a cure. Even when fully committed and engaged, biomedical institutions on the cutting edge of research prove themselves helpless before AIDS. Even though gay men are occasionally present as health-care workers, their tokenism does not wholly offset the homophobia gay men fear from the medical establishment. Despite all the efforts expended on Roger's behalf and all the lessons that might have been learned about his own illness, Monette does not expect that he himself will fare any better than Roger in finding help. Thus the opening line of the memoir ("I do not know if I will live to finish this") may be understood not only as a reflection on Monette's own mortality but also as a reflection on the state of medicine. Despite the structured efforts on the part of biomedical scientists to find a cure, there may never be a "magic bullet," even though the very pursuit of that objective fosters expectations of deliverance. Monette's memoir shows how medical promise can prove a receding, beckoning horizon that stays slightly beyond the hope it engenders in PWAs.

This treacherous kind of hope is somewhat tempered by an ambiguous effect of the search for a cure: the emergence of an AIDS underground. As Monette says of the band of gay men and PWAs looking for a cure:

This network has the feel of an underground railway. It could be argued that we're out there mainly for ourselves, of course, and the ones we cannot live without. But on the way we have also become traders and explorers, passing the word till hope is kindled in places so dark you can't see your hand in front of your eyes. If the government was going to act as if we didn't exist, if the medical establishment was prone to gridlock over funds, if the drug companies were waiting till the curve got high enough for profit, then we would find our own way.[29]

The AIDS underground functioned in part as a social form binding gay men together in ways that would not otherwise be possible in the shadow of homophobic medicine (and that would indeed not be required absent the epidemic). The search for a cure made some gay men more expert about AIDS early in the epidemic than most doctors, even in the most prestigious medical schools in the nation. Participation in a drug trial represented a willfulness to live that rang particularly strong in a culture whose medicine had declared "homosexuals" mentally ill and whose morality viewed homosexuality as ending in lonely, self-inflicted death. Anger at government and society at large and the search for an AIDS treatment at least had the effect of uniting PWAs in ways that served their own purposes. Monette's novel *Afterlife,* which followed *Borrowed Time,* continues this theme in showing how gay men and gay PWAs keep vigil over one another in homophobic society.[30]

In an implacable quest for an AIDS treatment, however, clinical drug trials and unorthodox treatments alike become overlaid with expectations that they could not possibly hope to meet. More important, their purposes may not be the purposes of individual PWAs. For example, even while suramin and AZT failed Roger, these failures are biomedical "successes" in the sense that they at least identify the limitations of those drugs as treatments. Even though they prove failures in saving individual lives, these kinds of "successes" can be as important to biomedical knowledge as clinical successes. Individuals may look to the advances of biomedical research for their individual salvation, but biomedical research need not save any given individual in order to advance itself. The AZT trial appears to have extended Roger's life for a time, and the search for a cure generated a camaraderie among the HIV infected that would not otherwise have been possible. There are reasons enough to acknowledge the worth of these advantages, but in the context of a health-care system that can be inimical to all patients and especially gay PWAs, even these advantages are not without their costs. How many times, after all, is a PWA supposed to want to survive the emergency hospitalizations, the intubations for mechanical ventilation, and the medications and sedation that are the treatment of *Pneumocystis* pneumonia? While biomedicine may benefit from putting PWAs through all these seemingly endless treatments in the sense that the pool of knowledge is thereby increased, still it is important not to mistake the needs of experimental research and the education of physicians for the needs of each individual PWA.

Medicine from the Garden Shed

David Wojnarowicz's "Living Close to the Knives" describes how his friend Peter Hujar, close to death and sicker all the time, explored various AIDS treatments. This memoir differs from Monette's in that its subject does not seek a cure in the halls of prestigious health centers. On the contrary, Peter gropes his way through unorthodox treatments. He had seen one researcher, for example, who had been working with "nontoxic antiviral drugs he'd developed." The researcher's investigations had elicited some sort of trouble with the federal government, but legal action failed to impugn the integrity or character of this particular researcher. In fact, action by a government discredited by its failure to appreciate the nature and magnitude of the epidemic actually *enhanced* his reputation: "The fact that the government entered the scene was one of the things that convinced Peter that the doctor might be a genius."[31] Part of the attraction here was the bold idea that the doctor had developed: injecting his patients with a "vaccine" made from human excrement.[32] Not even the fecal origin of this vaccine detracted from the doctor's credibility with his clients: "I figured that because shit was one of the most dangerous corporeal substances in terms of passing disease . . . maybe this guy figured out something in the properties of shit to develop a vaccine. After all, the bite of a rattlesnake is treated with a vaccine made of venom."[33] The doctor did fall from grace, however, when it was learned that only one person's excrement was the source of everyone's vaccine, that he covered up adverse reactions, and that he lied about how well others were doing ("fine, fine") when they were in fact sometimes dead and buried.

Wojnarowicz went next to a doctor on Long Island who was administering typhoid shots to PWAs on a theory that the injection somehow bolstered the immune system. Peter's raw emotions and disorientation beset the trip out to the doctor, but the encounter with the doctor proves more disconcerting still. The waiting room is full of familiar faces from the AIDS underground, fellow travelers recognizing one another from other waiting rooms, with a grapevine all their own. As in Monette's account, these cure seekers have assumed responsibility for their own treatment. One so-called "Dorian Gray," for example, both diagnoses and prescribes for himself, saying he won't need AL-721 because he only has AIDS-Related Complex, not AIDS.[34] In an ironic reversal of orthodox researchers' worries that their experiments will be disrupted by patients' taking unapproved drugs, other PWAs in the waiting room advise Peter to conceal his own use of AZT because this researcher wants to keep his unproven therapy uncontaminated by the confounding use of one of the drugs then formally licensed for the treatment of HIV infection![35]

The Long Island researcher opens up whole new possibilities of hope when he finally meets with Peter.[36] Ostensibly raising the question in the name of diagnostic certitude, the doctor asks Peter how he knows he has AIDS, adding, "After all, you may not have it." This question calls into doubt Peter's entire medical history and recasts his future. His "AIDS" might conceivably be cured by proving it never existed in the first place. The actual injection that Peter receives that day is an anticlimax to this more engaging possibility of deliverance. The narrator and another friend, however, are skeptical. Under their questioning, the "doctor" turns out to be "a research scientist with degrees in immunology" who offers them only a vague account of his theory connecting typhus injections with the thymus gland. They come away with their confidence in his medical knowledge significantly undercut. Neither the injection nor the prospect of correcting a misdiagnosis, however, proves of benefit; Peter dies later in the confines of an orthodox hospital, in keeping with his original orthodox diagnosis and prognosis.

Alternative medical treatment proves attractive for a number of reasons in this account.[37] Not only has Peter exhausted the routines and treatments available to him from orthodox medicine, but Wojnarowicz feels that orthodox medicine also stands as a figure for and is of a piece with the larger and morally corrupt society it serves. Wojnarowicz accuses the government of inaction and willful malfeasance toward PWAs. He notes, for example, how medicine's cultural distance from the sick and its general antipathy for gay men have forced PWAs to become not only their own researchers but also their own research subjects:

The government is not only witholding money, but drugs and information. People with AIDS across the country are turning themselves into human test tubes. Some of them are compiling so much information that they can call government agencies and pass themselves off as research scientists and suddenly have access to all the information that's been withheld and then they turn their tenement kitchens into laboratories, mixing up chemicals and passing them out freely to friends and strangers to help prolong lives. People are subjecting themselves to odd and sometimes dangerous alternative therapies—injections of viruses and consumption of certain chemicals used for gardening—all in order to live.[38]

While Wojnarowicz applauds the heroism in the efforts of PWAs to take matters into their own hands, he clearly does not find the cookery of alternative medicine any great consolation, given the brutal risks it entails and the larger social failing it represents. Wojnarowicz sees the therapeutic need created by AIDS as ultimately the responsibility of government and federal health agencies. Their failure to respond has turned PWAs by default into hobby researchers and kitchen chemists because they have no alternative.

Wojnarowicz connects Peter's death—and all deaths with AIDS—to the larger social hatred of gay men, to a homophobia and violence so pervasive that it both produces and sustains the ills of the epidemic. Given the willingness of people to blame PWAs for their illness and even a readiness to round them up in camps or to tattoo them, Wojnarowicz explains: "What's going on here but public and social murder on a daily basis and it's happening in our midst and not very many people seem to say or do anything about it."[39] The matter of rage at society is intimately connected with the search for an AIDS cure. In "X Rays from Hell," a tale that begins in a late afternoon conversation about the worth of living when, AZT notwithstanding, a friend's T-cells have plummeted to thirty, Wojnarowicz expresses this anger: "My rage is really about the fact that WHEN I WAS TOLD THAT I'D CONTRACTED THIS VIRUS IT DIDN'T TAKE ME LONG TO REALIZE THAT I'D CONTRACTED A DISEASED SOCIETY AS WELL."[40] He rejects the punishment theory of disease: that people die with AIDS because they have transgressed some moral norm or because they have internalized society's hatred of homosexuals.[41] He says, "I simply can't accept mystical answers or excuses for why so many people are dying from this disease—really it's on the shoulders of a bunch of bigoted creeps who at this point in time are in the position[s] of power that determine where and when and for whom government funds are spent for research and medical care."[42] AIDS here stands not only for the sickness set in motion by an HIV infection but as an indictment of pervasive and corrupt moral attitudes. A "cure" for AIDS therefore requires a much more broadly construed rescue than experimental pharmacology can by itself offer. Wojnarowicz observes:

Outside my windows there are thousands of people without homes who are trying to deal with having AIDS. If I think *my* life at times has a nightmarish quality about it because of the society in which I live and that society's almost total inability to deal with this disease with anything other than a conservative agenda, think for a moment what it would be like to be facing winter winds and shit menus at the limited shelters, and rampant TB, and the rapes, muggings, stabbings in those shelters, and the overwhelmed clinics and sometimes indifferent clinic doctors, and the fact that drug trials are not open to people of color or the poor unless they have a private physician who can monitor the experimental drugs they would need to take, and they don't have those kinds of doctors in clinics because doctors in clinics are constantly rotated and intravenous drug users have to be clean of drugs for seven years before they'll be considered for experimental drug trials, and yet there are nine-month waiting periods just to get assigned to a treatment program. So picture yourself with a couple of the three hundred and fifty opportunistic infections and unable to respond physiologically to the few drugs released by the foot-dragging deal-making FDA and having to maintain a junk habit; or even having to try and kick that habit without any clinical help while keeping yourself alive seven years to get a drug that you need immediately—thank you Ed Koch; thank you Stephen Joseph; thank you Frank Young; thank you AMA.[43]

Given Wojnarowicz's concern for the socially and medically disenfranchised, we are not surprised that he expresses so much interest in unorthodox medicine, even measuring its worth by the extent to which medical and governmental health agencies oppose it. At least unorthodox medicine will not be automatically tainted by complicity with these larger social failings.

As in other writing by gay men about the epidemic, Wojnarowicz's solution to the epidemic is intimately connected with greater access to drugs, government initiative in the development of treatment, and larger social reforms that work primarily to end homophobia but also to help the homeless, the poor, and the junkie PWAs. From this perspective a cure for AIDS cannot be limited to a pharmaceutical magic bullet that has as its only effect the control of HIV, for the oppressions of AIDS are more than the sum of their pathogenic parts. Even more than Monette, Wojnarowicz expresses a seething anger at the profound indifference of

American society to the lives of gay men and other disenfranchised minorities.

Orthodox medicine faces an important challenge in recognizing and responding to the meanings of AIDS in the lives of those whose economic and social situations do not permit them the luxury of monitoring the national AIDS grapevine for new drugs or checking themselves into comfortable hospitals for extended periods of experimental therapy. Even if medicine is on the road to the discovery of a cure for AIDS, the PWAs who inhabit Wojnarowicz's pages do not stand to benefit from it. Orthodox medicine not only fails to deliver what health-care services are available to all, it also fails to enroll PWAs in experimental anti-HIV drug trials. Drug-users and women, for example, generally face considerable obstacles in enrolling in drug trials.[44] Orthodox drug trials thereby become one of the problems facing socially disadvantaged PWAs of whatever sexual orientation. The "gold standard" of long-term, multisite, placebo-controlled testing, all carried out with the profit motive in mind, can prove no friend to the homeless PWA. By contrast, unorthodox treatments seem a kind of pharmaceutical lightning, which if it hits, may do so powerfully and memorably, but even Wojnarowicz's sympathetic account depicts the humiliating limits of alternative methods. Injections of shit into the bodies of PWAs serve as their own reductio ad absurdum.

Compassionate Access

Set in Paris, Hervé Guibert's *To the Friend Who Did Not Save My Life* is a thinly disguised account of Michel Foucault's death with AIDS and the author's own struggles with his HIV infection.[45] Professor of French literature Emily Apter rightly calls the work a mixed narrative form, neither fiction nor pure autobiography.[46] Foucault's longtime companion labeled the work a vicious fantasy, though it is clearly biographical in parts.[47] Sorting out what is and is not fictive in this account is not as important here as considering the encounters with medicine that dominate *To the Friend*. The portrait of medicine that emerges is anything but flattering. In fact, the narrative is a relentless account of the missteps, limitations, and duplicity of medicine. The account opens with a declaration that despite three months of despair, the narrator will prove one of the first survivors of AIDS. The author explains how his hopes are buoyed and sustained not by AZT or an underground treatment but by an "AIDS vaccine" coming from orthodox origins in American vaccine research. Yet in spite of the hope this vaccine inspires, *To the Friend* is largely an account of the way in which medicine fails people with AIDS.

Bill, an American manager of a large pharmaceutical lab that manufactures vaccines, is the first to tell the narrator (who stands for Guibert) in 1981 of a disease in the United States that is killing gay men. When the narrator passes this information along, his famous intellectual neighbor and friend, Muzil (who stands for Foucault), responds with incredulous laughter: "A cancer that would hit only homosexuals, no, that's too good to be true, I could just die laughing."[48] Ironically, Muzil will be among the first in France to die with the disease and among the most famous worldwide. His death in this narrative is made more ironic by his one-time encounter with a physician who hoped to establish dying centers where people could go and die quickly and painlessly, avoiding the long, revolting death agonies of hospices. Muzil had laughed this suggestion off too, though a version of this disappearing way of dying would prove attractive to him in his final days:

That nursing home of his, it shouldn't be a place where people go to die. Everything there should be luxurious, with fancy paintings and soothing music, but it would all be just camouflage for the real mystery, because there'd be a little door hidden away in a corner of the clinic, perhaps behind one of those dreamily exotic pictures, and to the torpid melody of a hypodermic nirvana, you'd secretly slip behind the painting, and presto, you'd vanish, quite dead in the eyes of the world, since no one would see you reappear on the other side of the wall, in the alley, with no baggage, no name, no nothing, forced to invent a new identity for yourself.[49]

This portrait of a vanishing, of a pretend death—taking the form, as the gravity of his illness became more apparent, of a wish to disappear in world travel—proves an ironic foil to Muzil's own all-too-corporeal death in the very hospital whose care of prostitutes and the insane Foucault had studied. There is precious little here to humanize Muzil's illness and death, and toward the end even such innocent trifles as pudding and copies of his new books were banished from his hospital room. The laughter that was Muzil's reaction to the first report of AIDS is transformed into a hacking cough that ends finally in his inability to speak. Before he died he knew full well how completely the body loses its identity once it is delivered into medical hands, "becoming just a package of helpless flesh, trundled around here and there, hardly even a number on a slip of paper, a name put through the administrative mill, drained of all individuality and dignity."[50]

There is some question in Foucault's own case of whether he knew or admitted to himself that he had been diagnosed with AIDS. Muzil's own expectations regarding diagnostic disclosure would permit him and others to avoid any unwanted information. In this regard Guibert reports Muzil as saying: "The doctor doesn't tell the patient the truth straight out, but he gives him the means and the opportunity, by talking in a roundabout way, to figure it out for himself, which also allows him to remain blessedly ignorant, if that's what he really wants."[51] The narrator does confront Muzil with the diagnosis of AIDS: "Actually, you hope you have AIDS." But Muzil "shot me a black look, one that brooked no appeal."[52] Even if Foucault knew that he had AIDS, there is still uncertainty about what he took it to mean. This uncertainty would at least have had the effect of staving off the doom associated by the media with the diagnosis in 1983 and 1984; there is even one point at which Muzil receives an astonishing declaration from a physician that he is in perfect health.[53] Not even this distancing of himself from AIDS, though, saves Muzil, who eventually dies under the reductive gaze and authority of medicine, all his expressed hopes for a death unattended by medicine thwarted, his death shadowed not only by the irony of his own earlier dismissal of a disease that stalks gay men but also by intimations that he knowingly participated in sex that might have infected others.[54]

The portrait of medicine that emerges in the course of the narrator's discovery of his own HIV infection paints medicine in castigating terms. Throughout this account there are all the predictable humiliations of patients, practically conventions of medicine, that are common in stories of sickness. Patients are kept waiting for unaccountable periods, they are left unattended during embarrassing and painful procedures and in unfriendly environments, and in one instance the narrator observes how his blood vials have been accidentally mixed up with those of another patient.[55] For his first blood tests, moreover, the narrator visited a clinic in an otherwise deserted and shuttered hospital on the verge of complete closure, the perfect cinematic symbol for medical desolation. Elsewhere in the account, physicians are rebuked for improprieties. One doctor insisted on an HIV test the narrator did not want.[56] Another put the narrator at risk of liver cancer through mismanagement of hepatitis.[57] Another gossiped indiscreetly about his patients.[58] A homeopath diagnosed the narrator's throat abscess as "spasmophilia," a semivoluntary condition caused by a lack of calcium, something requiring the "treatment" of mineral water and lemon.[59] That same doctor treated female patients by "shutting them up nude inside metal chests after affixing needles all over their bodies, needles filled with concentrates made from herbs, tomatoes, bauxite, pineapples, cinnamon, patchouli, turnips, clay, and carrots . . ."[60] Yet another doctor diagnosed Guibert as suffering from "dysmorphophobia," a hatred of all forms of deformity.[61] A psychiatrist challenges a patient to admit that his AIDS is the culmination of his own longing for death.[62] So harsh and humiliating are Guibert's encounters with medicine here and in his subsequent book that Emily Apter has called his work a "tragicomic version of *La Ronde,* in which doctors, visited in rapid succession and submitted to without a word, are substituted for the tricks of old."[63]

While the narrator's emotions are infused with hope for treatment of his HIV infection, his search for a vaccine parallels the kind of willful submission to mortification which is typical of masochism. The term *vaccine* is used by Guibert, as it has been used by Jonas Salk and others, to describe a treatment used on persons already infected with HIV which introduces some altered and nonpathogenic form of HIV in order to evoke an immune response capable of acting against pathogenic HIV. Such a treatment could then be administered prophylactically to others not yet infected. Bill, an American pharmaceutical executive, describes the possibility of a trial of such a vaccine in France and it becomes the narrator's sustaining hope. At the very same time Dr. Chandi invites the narrator to participate in a double-blind, placebo-controlled drug trial. This kind of trial meets the scientific community's requirement of ruling out the psychologically powerful placebo effect (in which the mere expectation of benefit from a drug produces the benefit sought). The pretense of placebos is found repugnant by the narrator ("abominable, real torture for all the patients involved"[64]) and all the more so when he discovers that Dr. Chandi had lied to him. Dr. Chandi admitted that "he was already convinced at that time that the real medication was as useless as the dummy." It was only at the insistence of the pharmaceutical company that physicians continued to seek subjects for the study.[65]

After his formal diagnosis of HIV and his refusal to participate in Dr. Chandi's drug study, the narrator's T-cell count starts to fall, and it appears that his only option is AZT. But even if the AZT is successful in sustaining his life, it will entail lifelong dependency and pose such side effects as nausea, vomiting, headache, skin rash, stomachache, muscular pain, insomnia, intense fatigue, diarrhea, dizziness, and taste disorders.

Against this background the narrator listens in awe to Bill's description of the vaccine. But the hope held out by the vaccine—months away at best—is still no reason for unalloyed optimism. As Guibert puts it: "Now I was entering a new phase, a limbo of hope and uncertainty, that was perhaps more terrible to live through than the one before."[66] The personal treachery that follows justifies this description. Bill had promised to find a way to put the narrator (and companions Jules and Berthe) in the French trial, making sure they did not get placed in the placebo arm. Bill even went so far as to say that he would take the group to the United States and have the vaccine's creator vaccinate them if necessary.[67] Bill proves, however, unfaithful and unreliable, and all his many promises do not lead to the vaccine. He does, however, find a way to put another friend in the trial. This outcome should not have been too surprising; the narrator himself notes how hard it had been to secure a ride home with Bill. The very scarcity of the vaccine trial slots opened the narrator and his companions to manipulation. The "science" of biomedical research proves itself again susceptible to human vice, in this case favoritism, a bias that may not work against the results necessary for science but that surely works against the interests of the narrator, who looks to biomedicine for his very survival. This favoritism even deranges what camaraderie is possible between gay men in the epidemic.

As in Monette's writing, Guibert's narrative pitches PWAs into a maelstrom of conflicting opinion even as they are forced to acquire what expertise is possible on AIDS. Guibert's narrator finds himself trapped, for example, between conflicting opinions on how much AZT to take, opinions from two equally credible physicians offering equally credible rationales for their dosage recommendations.[68] The scene is a medical reenactment of the paradox of Buridan's ass: situated equally distant from two identical and equally attainable bales of hay, unable to identify any advantage in one over the other and therefore unable to choose between them, the ass starves to death. In such circumstances when all medication options appear equally limited, the prospect of an AIDS vaccine did offset psychologically the symptoms Guibert was enduring, fatigue and thrush among them. But the lure of a vaccine also and more importantly offered shelter from the responsibility for decisions about medication and offered the appearance of medicine more attentive to human needs and less wracked by the vagaries of conflicting scientific opinion.

There are instances in Guibert's narrative in which he pursues medical and emotional certainty another way. After examination by one particularly unorthodox doctor, the narrator says, "I'll kiss the hand of the person who'll tell me I'm doomed."[69] Or again, he says, "I felt better the moment I learned I had AIDS."[70] "If Bill were to file an appeal against my death sentence with his vaccine, he'd plunge me back into my former state of ignorance. [The diagnosis of] AIDS has enabled me to make a huge breakthrough in my life."[71] Even as he anticipates the possibility of the vaccine, his commitment wanes: "But [Bill] was tired, and so was I, and it was as though neither of us believed anymore in the possibility of this vaccine and its power to bring my disease under control, as though, in the end, languidly, we no longer gave a damn, just didn't give a fucking damn."[72] Or again, the narrator imagines Bill stealing the vaccine and crashing with it into the Atlantic.[73] Whatever else these declarations might reveal about the psychology of the narrator, they show how the anticipation of death can offer a repose incompatible with the demonic stalking of the ever-new offerings of medicine. Guibert's narrative demonstrates how the pursuit of a cure requires that hope submit—as a condition of its very possibility—to endless medical scrutiny and experimentation, the brusqueness of physicians, and the venality of pharmaceutical executives.

Although the book opens on a note of optimism and commitment to being among the first survivors of AIDS, the narrator's final medical decision is to discontinue AZT. He ends his book saying: "I'm in deep shit. Just how deep do you want me to sink? Fuck you, Bill! My muscles have melted away. At last my arms and legs are once again as slender as they were when I was a child."[74] The failures of medicine in this account are often personal ones, belonging to specific physicians, nurses, and Bill especially. But the narrator's indictment—"In Bill's eyes, I'm already dead"[75]—encompasses the practitioners, the institutions, and the principles of medicine alike, if not for their outright abandonment of PWAs then at least for the way medicine can—in the guise of helping them—actually flog people with HIV toward their deaths.

The Cost of a Cure

Placebo means in Latin "I will please." Clinical drug and surgical trials attempt to isolate and extinguish any outcome that depends on the placebo effect, the improvement based on the expectation of benefit by the experimental subject. But as the chronicles discussed above indicate, many more "pleasures" are extinguished in medicine besides those that confound experimentation. In their chronicles of the search for an AIDS treatment Monette, Wojnarowicz, and Guibert try to reintroduce important pleasures of PWAs back into medicine. Their search for an AIDS cure almost starts from the assumption that medicine is no antagonist to their pleasures, especially the pleasure of individual recovery from AIDS. Their own accounts, however, do not always support the uncritical fervency with which they pursue a cure for AIDS.

These authors do not confine their expectations of medicine to their own isolated hopes of healing. In their narratives the hope for an effective AIDS treatment is virtually indistinguishable from expectations about biomedical reform generally, and if their narratives are read as indictments they fault not only individual practitioners for harsh treatment but also the institutional values of medicine as prejudicial to gay men and those in need of experimental medicine. Nevertheless, Monette, Wojnarowicz, and Guibert all seem to believe that the march of biomedicine cannot but produce a cure, and this view is shared by others in AIDS activism as well. The operational assumption of Larry Kramer, for example, is that a cure for AIDS exists and that it is merely necessary to find it; in his analysis finding a cure means getting past the homophobia, bureaucratic intransigence, and political incompetence that keep medicine from doing its job.[76] Cinema historian and AIDS activist Vito Russo also proclaimed that one day the AIDS crisis will be over.[77] But perhaps unwittingly and contrary to their intentions Monette, Wojnarowicz, and Guibert make it clear that advances toward a cure are paid for in the currency of the suffering of people with AIDS. More often than not, a diagnosis of AIDS sets in motion a litany of examinations, tests, hospitalizations, and desperate fumblings in the realm of alternative medicine.

I do not wish to say that PWAs or any other group of persons suffering from illness ought not to pursue treatment and cures even if it falls to them to become experts about their conditions and prove the moral conscience for medicine. But I do wonder whether advocates of an unyielding belief in a cure for AIDS and a demand for that cure don't underappreciate the damaging effects of medical care and research. It is worth asking whether the search for a cure is modeling itself on a relentless consumerism, with the pursuit of experimental drugs taking its place alongside the Jaguar, the hillside home with pool, the imported goods, and the other amenities of upscale urban living as the symbols of a fulfilling life. We may also ask in light of the narratives considered above to what extent the despair of PWAs can actually be an artifact of misplaced faith in the very capacities of biomedicine. Activist demands for an AIDS treatment come at a time when other social and legal forces are converging to secure ways of protecting patients from unwanted, ineffective, and sometimes brutalizing medical treatment. The federal Patient Self-Determination Act, for example, was prompted in part by the desire to protect patients from the damages of unrestrained medical treatment,[78] and the death-delivering "Mercitron" of Jack Kevorkian and the thanatological recipes of Derek Humphrey's *Final Exit* have adherents of their own among the sick and dying.[79]

In 1993 the Ninth International AIDS Conference in Berlin ended in pessimism about the prospect for early development of a prophylactic HIV vaccine, and its reports cast a long shadow over the efficacy of AZT, the most widely used drug for treatment of people with HIV-related disease. Conference presenters and reports associated this pessimism with the slow nature of science rather than with the nature of HIV.[80] One may read this kind of pessimism in the same way that the 1993 National Research Council Report on AIDS[81] can be read: as the predictable reeling in of a decade of outlandish discourse on the future of AIDS. After all, immunological prosperity was said to be around the corner more than once. One need only recall Secretary of Health and Human Services Margaret Heckler's overweening declaration in 1984 that a vaccine for what was then called HTLV-III was only two years away.[82] Or one might read the somber, circumspect reports from the Berlin conference as evidence of waning social and medical commitment to the cause of discovering a cure. Either way, the conference functioned as a biomedical echo of these turn-of-the-decade narratives by Monette, Wojnarowicz, and Guibert about the results of a committed search for an AIDS treatment: all heroic efforts notwithstanding, there is no curative treatment for the pathogenesis of HIV infection, and none is on the horizon.

The enormity of the task of finding a cure for AIDS permits raising the question of moral responsibility in that task. Certainly people with severe illnesses want to discover a treatment that will restore them to health, and certainly society should invest in therapies and research. But it is hard to see that a morally defensible argument could maintain that PWAs and others with incurable conditions are individually duty-bound to discover a cure. It is also hard to see that any PWA has the duty to be the first person whose AIDS is cured. AIDS activism committed to the demand for an immediate cure sets the threshold for "responsible" living with AIDS higher than would seem to be justified in terms of a person's moral duties. If, as Larry Kramer says, a cure for AIDS exists and merely needs to be discovered, it is easy to see PWAs and society at large as amiss if they do not pursue that cure with every effort that can be mustered. But such a judgment is unreasonable given the distance that appears to separate PWAs from a cure. If, moreover, one assumes that governmentally coordinated medicine may identify a cure for AIDS, one may wonder by extension whether similar efforts could not also identify cures for many other conditions. To the extent human disorders are the result of identifiable biological processes open to human intervention and control, in theory a cure would exist for all such human suffering. If so, there are more failures than successes in medicine, and to the extent these failures belong to human action and indecision the government not only has blood on its hands but buckets and buckets of it.

A cure for AIDS is important, yes, but it does not follow that each and every PWA must commit to the pursuit of that cure as if it were the only morally permissible objective for him or her. Since the task of finding a cure appears more and not less daunting with every passing international AIDS conference, it is well to keep in mind the dangers of overcommitment to a goal whose pursuit appears to be largely a matter of supererogation, of individual willingness to tolerate the limitations and disappointments of medicine. There is every reason to pursue treatment and a cure, but not a cure that imperils the other values important to PWAs. Recognition of the dangers posed by medicine to PWAs is not incompatible with views advocating stronger social investment in efforts to care for PWAs in all their needs. In extending the dominion of medicine over the cruelties of nature, the search for a cure affirms the worth of PWAs and the importance of human knowledge. But the pursuit of an AIDS cure, if it is swollen beyond reason, may prove as defeating as utter resignation to the inevitability of death with AIDS. In a review of Hervé Guibert's *To the Friend Who Did Not Save My Life*, gay novelist and essayist Andrew Holleran observed: "As the deaths increase in number, and the dead become more various, the recriminations are going to mount. In the broadest sense, everyone who survives did not save the lives of those who didn't."[83] A cure for AIDS, envisioned as involving the rehabilitation of medical research, the eradication of homophobia, and the humanization of medical practice, is certainly attractive in its revolutionary ambitions. At the same time, though, Holleran's remark can be interpreted to suggest that uncritical insistence on a cure risks expanding the breadth of human moral depravity to the point where mere survival amounts to complicity in others' deaths with AIDS. Surely the search for treatment and a cure should not have to incriminate every innocent of every human life and stoke every rage against dying when death can sometimes offer the sick more consolations than medicine.

3

Testimony

The writing about the experience of sickness and death in the AIDS epidemic, much of it by and about gay men, comes on the heels of the rise of noteworthy gay literature in the United States. Richard Hall has drawn attention to some of the ways that literature has changed considerably since World War II. What was once a literature of secrecy, guilt, and apology has become a literature of defiance and celebration of sexual difference, a literature offering characters who are gay without complaint: "No more slashed wrists and leaps into the sea."[1] Such characters are no longer typically enmeshed in psychiatric and moral quagmires by reason of their homoerotic lives; they have escaped definition by social stigmas, and they resist the distortion of their private truths by public mythology.

Gay and lesbian literature now charts the familiar problems of looking for love, finding a family, determining the worth of career and power in the order of things.[2] In moving to concerns about relationships and families, gay literature has had to move beyond coming-out stories in order to address the trials of ordinary human life, love gone wrong, and the aging and death of parents. And such a literature has also had to countenance the HIV/AIDS epidemic and grapple not only with unexpected illness and death but also with its moral and cultural meanings.

This writing has taken various forms in fiction, poetry, biography, autobiography, and even obituaries. Obituaries are now as much a standard feature of the pages of the *Windy City Times*, the *Advocate*, and the *New York Native* as their inevitable phone-sex ads. In obituary form or otherwise, much of this writing has taken as its task the blessing of the dead. Of course, not only gay men have written about their experiences and losses in the epidemic. Other people close to the devastations of AIDS and its antecedents in HIV infection have also set down their encounters with illness, dying, loss, and fear. But on the whole, there are precious few encomiums penned to poor, drug-using men and women who have died with AIDS. Gay men, either as author or subject, dominate the written word in the literature of the epidemic. Their publications and booksellers are the epicenters of writing about AIDS.

Douglas Crimp has said, *"Anything said or done about AIDS that does not give precedence to the knowledge, the needs, and the demands of people living with AIDS must be condemned."*[3] Taken literally, this position condemns the worth of writing about those sick or dead with AIDS unless that writing also serves in a utilitarian way the cause of those with AIDS who remain behind. But this would be a stern requirement imposed on those who want, whatever else they want to do with their writing, to testify to the worth and value of those persons who have died. Writing about the dead may or may not have explicit activist dimensions—some writing does certainly involve explicit and implicit political critique—but to declare such writing worthwhile only insofar as it advances a political or medical reformation is to deny its own inherent moral integrity. In fact, Crimp himself has come to conjoin rather than detach mourning and militancy.[4] Elegiac writing does not say all that needs to be said in the epidemic and it may be sometimes a poor substitute for informed and effective political discourse. But it is better to write something than to say nothing and thereby let death in its extinguishing finality arrogate to itself all privilege in deciding the fate and worth of human life. Elegy, or testimony, as I prefer to call it, belongs to the continuum of moral and political conscience which fuels activism in the epidemic and has an important function in the protection of the individual.[5] Such testimony also offers the opportunity for resisting the infantilizing of the dying and the dead which often occurs in the context of their health care. The moral and political dimensions of elegies and their insistence on the primacy of the individual are evident in representative examples from the literature of testimony.

The Testimonials

Barbara Peabody was among the very first to chronicle in journal form her experiences in caring for her son, sick and dying with AIDS. In *The Screaming Room*[6] she describes how her gay son, Peter VonLehn, aspired to a career in opera and theater but worked mostly as a waiter in New York. She remembers him as bright, inquisitive, musical, introspective, intellectual, imaginative, humorous, and independent. After being diagnosed with AIDS in December 1983, Peter returned from New York to live with his mother in San Diego. Peabody tells of tending her son on the good days and the bad. In this account small events loom large against the confines and constraints of Peter's illness; as a result, her story has much in common with the often slow, tedious, and oppressive narratives of prison life. There were sleepless nights and intractable diarrhea, reclusive behavior and loss of memory, endless trips to doctors and hospitals, spinal taps and drug regimens, the loss of sight, and finally the watch at the deathbed. There is pain and suffering on every page of this book. At Peter's death there is nothing left for Peabody but tears: "I am just another mother who has lost her child, who holds his empty, wasted body in her arms and mourns, grieves, cries for loss of part of her own body and soul."[7] But for all the suffering, for all the costs she paid in caring for him, the book remains nevertheless a memorial to Peter and to her love of him. And despite the suffering they both endured, she never hoped for his death.

Andrew Holleran's novel *Dancer from the Dance* appeared in the late seventies and told the tale of drag queen Sutherland and his handsome protégé Malone as they spent their lives looking for love in Manhattan's nights, discos, parks, and bathhouses, at summer parties in the Pines, in drugs, in any pair of eyes, really, that offered a promise of repose. Instead, now, of stories about long nights, extravagant parties, and the art of cruising which were integral to his *Dancer* and the later *Nights in Aruba*,[8] Holleran writes mostly about the consequences of the HIV epidemic, about hospitals and funerals, about the deeply felt loss of friends, about the loss of the period he described in his haunting first novel, a period that looks to be gone forever, felled by the most archaic form of life, a virus. Nostalgia permeates these essays, which continue to appear in *Christopher Street*, nostalgia for the forms of intimacy and belonging which the epidemic has closed off to gay men.

Holleran also offers reflections on the all too many men in his circle who have died. There is a remembrance of Cosmo, thus nicknamed for his worldly air.[9] He and Holleran became friends in Philadelphia. Cosmo had a mania for puns as well as a wicked sense of humor. "He seemed, on his ten-speed with his knapsack, utterly independent, as if all he needed in life was a combination lock, a Penguin paperback, and a can of V-8 juice." After a separation of a few years, Holleran dialed Cosmo's number only to be told that Cosmo was dead with AIDS. "Cosmo was not like everyone else," Holleran says, "Cosmo was special." "Cosmo loved life, treasured his body, was only thirty-five, succeeded in his career, and had much to look forward to." Holleran is grieved to observe that despite the death of a person so much to be treasured that New York and the world at large could proceed as if Cosmo were utterly dispensable. *The New York Times* would continue to make its daily report and Chernobyl's radioactive cloud would spread westward across Europe as if there had never been a Cosmo. Though Holleran had already experienced other deaths with AIDS and knew as well as anyone that everyone dies, still he was shattered by the inexplicable death: "Cosmo's death horrified. What a waste! What an insult!" No theory could make sense of the death as a moral judgment, as the consequence of self-hate, the inability to love, or even shame at being gay: "His death does not illuminate anything that leaves us morally edified, or superior, or enlightened—it was just part of the vast human waste that is occurring; just mean and nasty."

Holleran also remembers Ernie Mickler, author of the well-known *White Trash Cooking*. Holleran points out that Ernie was funny, had high spirits, nerve, wit, style, and stories to tell. Mickler planned the details of his funeral down to the menu to be served at the luncheon afterward, and Holleran finds himself feeling helpless at not being able to thank his friend for this last kindness. He finds the world emptier without Ernie even as the world seems to bespeak his presence: "The day is hazy and warm, the river flat and still, the woods soft and empty, and the whole afternoon, somehow, like the lunch itself, part of Ernie."[10] Holleran also recalls Eddie, whose life Holleran found essential to the vitality of New York. Eddie lived nocturnally, was in the clubs almost every night, knew the details of New York, knew where to get a Shiatsu massage, to buy cowboy boots, to see a strip show near Times Square. Eddie unfailingly enjoyed everything new in the city: nightclubs, phone systems, winter coats. Holleran has the impression that Eddie got AIDS only because, ironically, he was the first to do everything. After Eddie's death, Holleran finds, the city is less vital even as, somehow, Eddie remains present in spite of his death.[11] This refrain recurs in much writing about people who have died with AIDS: death does not extinguish personal presence. On the contrary, death and absence may confirm its very existence and importance.

Holleran writes about many more deaths besides. There was the death of Charles Ludlam, the founder of the Ridiculous Theater Company. Holleran is lavish in his praise here: Ludlam was actor, playwright, genius, anarchist, madman. He was loony as Rasputin and funny beyond accounting.[12] There is also a reflection on O., sick with AIDS, less known to the world but worldly nevertheless, especially as a host par excellence. Facing O.'s likely death, Holleran wonders how it is possible to thank him for the many years of wit, wine, conversation, laughter, happiness. How is it possible to make sense of so substantial a man laid waste by this disease?[13] There is an account of Michael, who came from a good family, went to Cornell, kept a garden, was a talented architect, and, before the sickness, was concupiscent and lascivious. What, Holleran wonders, did the germs need with him?[14] In tracing the swath of death through his friends, Holleran also memorializes the late George Stambolian, professor at Wellesley College and editor of the well-regarded *Men on Men* collections, as "handsome in a way faces were handsome hundreds of years ago, in Byzantium."[15] As the dying is not over yet, one may suppose that Holleran will offer more memorials as there comes more death day after day, name after name, without end in sight. Such portraits as these put a face on the epidemic and offer a counterliterature to the discourse of medical journals where PWAs are described as patients or cases or to the discourse of the media where PWAs are still described and represented as victims and predators. These testimonials certainly give the lie to the notion that PWAs are beyond the moral community—are both unloving and unloved. Such portraits may not always "analyze" the broad cultural assumptions which encase the epidemic, but they do identify those in whose name analysis and activism go forward. One could not, after all, find Peter VonLehn or Eddie Mickler when looking at the numbers in the latest edition of the *HIV/AIDS Surveillance Report* from the Centers for Disease Control. As a mere assortment of diagnoses and treatments their medical charts would also be unrevealing. If there is a counter-discourse to the stereotyping and stigmatizing uses of "AIDS," it must begin with the names and lives of those who have borne the burden of the epidemic.

Testimony and Its Meanings

AIDS incites the impulse to memorialize, but that impulse is not uniform in its purposes or forms. The meanings of testimonial range from verbal portraiture to personal healing to examination of the meaning of sickness and death in the order of human life. Its methods range from ceremonious hagiography to self-conscious wit. The methods and styles of testimony often converge as acts of memory about the lives of the dead, and it is worth examining testimony's form and content to assess what those acts are understood to mean. Testimonial writing first creates a record of the lives of the dead, sharing details beyond name, age, and residence. Such writing often attempts to approximate—to the extent this is possible—a verbal equivalent of the presence of the dead. Yet writing is no substitute for the dead themselves, and their loss—a loss that cannot be recompensed—leaves authors like Holleran looking for answers about the meaning of the epidemic, of life itself. What can it all mean that these men suffer and die? What can all the beauty and intimacy of men be for if not to live and love in the ways they can? What can all the virtue and accomplishment of life mean if they die nonetheless?[16] If, as Holleran's writing seems to suggest, the world does not care about the dead, there are still those who do care when they write and those who do when they read testimonials. Thus is this writing also a protest at what happens to mortal beings.

This is not to say that these pieces have been written only as eulogy. Most authors of these accounts say that they have written for other reasons as well: Many speak of the need to make sense of events. Peabody said she wrote to fend off grief: "I gradually found my way out of my screaming room by sorting out and writing down all that happened to us."[17] Elizabeth Cox says that she wrote *Thanksgiving*, recounting her husband's death with AIDS, to create something that would help her remember, make sense of the unexplainable, and give her a place to put the anger she felt at the cruelty of life. Andrew Holleran has said too that writing offers a way of coping with adversity, even if only to probe the questions forced by unexpected death.[18] Paul Monette offers the same motive: writing offers a small measure of power over the nightmare.[19] Much of the writing about those with HIV-related conditions also details the considerable efforts exerted by family and friends to secure help and comfort for the sick and the dying.[20]

Testimonial writing also seems to offer some measure of healing—and this is not an inconsequential good. Such writing is not typically, however, mired in its own solipsistic needs. Writers like Peabody and Holleran frequently express the hope that others will not have to go through such trials, that the epidemic will be brought to an end. Although these authors may begin with private grief, many of them consciously aim beyond the limits of personal anguish and, in articulating the need for the conquest of the epidemic, do not mistake profound sorrow as any substitute for education and social action. Without judging the extent to which she may have been successful in this regard, Elizabeth Cox says, for example, that she wrote to help overcome social ignorance and indifference to AIDS.[21] Even if testimonial writing begins as so much flailing at unbearable emotions, it nevertheless can heal and can have the effect of making it easier for others to talk about AIDS—easier for others, whatever their political, sexual, and cultural agenda, to care about the epidemic.

Borrowed Time remains the most accomplished memoir to appear in English thus far. There Paul Monette discusses the life and loss of his friend and lover, Roger Horwitz. Monette has also written about their relationship and the place of AIDS in it in a collection of poems, *Love Alone*.[22] Paul and Roger met at a party on Boston's Beacon Hill and were lovers for over twelve years, not without difficulties, not either without sex outside the relationship. Roger was diagnosed with AIDS in March 1985 and died in October of the following year. Monette himself also has the HIV-related disease: "The virus ticks in me."[23]

Roger's illness began as minor frets—the loss of a few pounds, minor coughing, short periods of fever, nothing really that made either of them think of AIDS—and ended in a broad array of debilitating disorders: bouts of *Pneumocystis carinii* pneumonia, thrush, herpes, kidney disorder, blindness, shingles, and more. Like Peabody before him, Monette tells about shuttling Roger to doctors, about experimental drugs, about all the kinds of care Roger needed, about the worries and concerns of friends and family, about watching others in their circle of friends fall ill and die after diagnoses of AIDS. Monette protects Roger in the ways that he can: providing the right food, dousing him with vitamins, steering him clear of dirt, cautioning against strain, berating neighbors for the overflow of their septic tank.

Monette offers unreserved praise for Roger throughout the memoir:

> How do I speak of the person who was my life's best reason? The most completely unpretentious man I ever met, modest and decent to such a degree that he seemed to release what was most real in everyone he knew. It was always a relief to be with Roger, not to have to play any games at all. By a safe mile he was the least flashy of all our bright circle of friends, but he spoke about books and the wide world he had journeyed with huge conviction and a hunger to know everything.[24]

Monette, moreover, even characterizes Roger as a paradigm of the classical Greek ideal of virtue, *sophrosyne:* the whole of virtue characterized by a harmony of soul acting according to right reason. He lavishes praise and celebrates Roger's native intellect, his commitment and devotion in their relationship, and his endurance throughout the nineteen-month course of illness. When Monette's own disturbingly low T-cell counts came rolling in, Roger was there, says Monette, with loyalty and concern.[25] Even in the worst throes of illness, Monette credits Roger with always looking on the bright side.[26] He is hard pressed to understand why Roger does not cry out against his blindness.[27] It is, Monette thinks, as if Roger had an instinct to make others feel better.[28]

Monette does not try to resurrect Roger with this memoir; nor does he mistake writing for taxidermy. It is not Roger's life that Monette is trying to hold onto here, it is his *goodness.* And the incentive for that effort is nothing more than the finitude of human life resisted by the counsels of human love. "Loss teaches you very fast," Monette says, "what you cannot go without saying."[29] Disease may kill, but it cannot always diminish the importance of a single human life, cannot always silence the voice of tribute. The line between praise of the dead and protest against death is a slim one indeed.

Narratives about those dead with AIDS typically praise the worth of the dead, citing variously their interests and their contributions. They speak of love of travel and cooking, attachment to friends and family, affection for pets, passion in politics, accomplishments of intellect, and madcap senses of humor. In this regard obituaries in the gay press are often more indulgent than those in mass-circulation papers. Such obituaries may describe in some detail the persons who have died with AIDS and their influence on the circle of people who loved them. Any one obituary chosen at random from, say, the *PWA Newsline* shows considerable effort at sympathetic portraiture. For example, in describing John B. Hettwer, an artist and dancer, his lover Stephen describes him as "a striking vision of compact muscular power and physical beauty with crystal blue eyes and a golden halo of hair. He was the most generous and kind person I have ever known. His smile spoke of a warm heart, a great sense of humor, [a] sexy and confident young man of strong opinion and honest conscience."[30]

Testimonial writing does not necessarily blink away individual failings. Barbara Peabody was aware of certain failings of her son, seeing in his character the weakness that put him in the path of HIV infection; she thought him impetuous and self-destructive and inattentive to his native gifts.[31] In *Borrowed Time* Monette likewise expresses his anger at Roger for getting sick: "My anger was growing more and more unmanageable. But I thought I understood the difference—then, anyway—between being mad at him and being mad at AIDS."[32] Elizabeth Cox also reports a great deal of anger toward her husband when she discovered his relationships with men.[33] Yet in the end anger was either a luxury made impossible by the demands of caring for the sick or it was beside the point.

It may be surprising that so many sins are forgiven and vices forgotten in writing about the dead. The living we often judge unsparingly. Why do the dead escape our harsh judgments when they can no longer exert any form of resistance or revenge? Why does vice wither away without a trace in the grave? In the end, for example, Elizabeth Cox does not dwell on the way her husband may have put her and their son at risk of HIV infection. There are no angry remonstrances in *Borrowed Time* about whose sexual liaisons might have been responsible for whose infection. Perhaps such forgiveness is itself an act of compassion, a way of making amends for the evil suffered in death. Silence about vices is perhaps a way of saying that no evil deserves the consequence of death or that in death there is already what punishment any theory of retribution could require.

In their spoken and unspoken meanings obituaries and other first-person accounts of the dead have much in common with the appliqué panels of the Names Project.[34] However else they might be interpreted, the panels can be seen as soft-sculpture tombstones whose display, for example, on the Capitol Mall in the District of Columbia, evokes a cemetery in visual expanse and moral purpose. The panels themselves are sometimes beautiful, witty, poignant, and funny. Even when they are simple and artless, they are motivated by a desire to name and preserve the significance of the person who has died and to honor if not assuage the loss felt by those left behind. Letters often accompany these panels as they come into the headquarters of the Names Project. Often simple and always sad, these letters written by lovers, friends, mothers, fathers, sisters, brothers, and even strangers explain how they have come to make the panel they are submitting. They describe the persons with AIDS in an endless catalog of virtues: talented, special, courageous, compassionate, loyal, dedicated, encouraging, original, honest, kind, helpful, warm, gentle, motivating, confident, assured, artistic, funny, intelligent. The letters and panels make it clear that they seek to preserve the memory of a life that touched them, that deserves something better than silence.

The attempt to point out individual virtues is an archetypal feature of writing about the dead. Assertions of love, of worth, and of loss are universal. Some descriptions raise the religious belief of an afterlife in order to hope the dead will go on living, their virtues intact for all eternity. And it is interesting that the chief value perceived in that afterlife is not typically union with God and the glory of that experience but the chance to see human friends and loved ones again, which says as much about the origin of heaven as any other account. A hope of this kind is an assertion that one cannot be alone in the universe, that there must be something at the center of being that impels human lives toward their happiness, that people cannot live with others and love them only to have them turn to dust. Not all persons, of course, share such a religious belief, and for those who do not, death is that much more a tragedy without recompense. But what consolations there may be are nevertheless found and asserted: the time shared together, the hope that one person's struggle with AIDS will help spare others in the future or that a life's influence will continue to be felt even long after death.

Testimonials almost always protest that those who have died with AIDS have died too early, too young, with too many things undone. Implicit in such a view is the notion that death is less an atrocity if it comes later in life. Perhaps aging is after all a consolation in the way it prepares us for death by withering our bodies, minds, and even our hopes. But perhaps this is the rationalization of inevitability. If senescence were a disorder inflicted on us involuntarily by another person or caused by a communicable virus, it would be intolerable: we would condemn it outright as an immorality of the first order. Perhaps, then, we need to wonder if aging and death are any less an atrocity because they come from nature. Perhaps we need to wonder if illness, death, and grief teach us anything that we do not already know many times over.

Could it be that all death—and not only death with AIDS—is always an atrocity? That the origins of medicine are to be found in its protest? Barring any breakthrough that could stave off aging and death, we are left of course to countenance the lives we must have. In the circumstances in which we live, the years are precious enough, writers about the unexpected dead seem to say, that not even one can be spared.

There is much solemnity in elegiac tributes to the dead. Funerary rituals—obituaries, funerals, religious services—invite such responses. This very chapter has observed a grave tone. Given the link posited between humor to aggression, no one is surprised that on occasions of sickness and death humor is set aside in favor of dignified discourse. But humor and wit also represent resilient energy and strength and these forms break through in testimonials as well. The "'zine" *Diseased Pariah News* appropriates its name from a cultural perception of people with HIV and serves as "a forum for infected people to share their thoughts, feelings, art, writing, and brownie recipes in an atmosphere free of teddy bears, magic rocks, and seronegative guilt."[35] That desktop publication treated the death of one of its founders satirically, showing on its cover an immolated teddy bear: "Darn!" read the accompanying headline, "One of our editors is dead!" Such satirical treatment and the coupling of wit with grief do not deny the importance of death, but neither do they submit tamely to the formalism of funereal forms and cheap sentiment, and they permit expressions of strength and resilience even in the face of the epidemic. Thus is to be explained the possibility of laughter in the epidemic.[36] Laughter and not only rage function as refutation of worthlessness in the epidemic. Laughter as much as tears can affirm the worth of the dead.

Obituaries and Activism

For all the good intentions at work in memorializing, writing about the dead sometimes risks sentimental self-indulgence. It is, after all, easy to find in another's death evidence of one's own good fortune and moral nobility. The effort exerted on behalf of writing may seem, moreover, ill-justified when printed pages do not take anyone out of a hospital bed. In "Reading and Writing," Holleran says he cannot imagine anyone reading books about AIDS with pleasure. The only thing people want to read, he suggests, is the headline: CURE FOUND. How can one write when the suffering is so real? when all that matters is taking care of friends, starting support services, and carrying out the lab work that can bring all the misery to a hasty conclusion? Writing is helpless, he says, because it cannot produce a cure, it cannot heal, and it cannot explain. The best writing, he predicts, may likely turn out to be a lament that we are as flies to wanton gods killing us for their sport or a simple list of names—those who behaved well, those who behaved badly in the epidemic.[37] Nonetheless, he acknowledges, one must continue to write if only to relieve anxiety and depression.

Other good reasons exist as well. Thus are to be explained the many AIDS volumes and articles on cultural criticism, social policy, legal analysis, medical research, and other topics yet to be considered. This wealth of motives and forms of narrative about the sick and the dead show that writing is not always an idle extravagance. On the contrary, such writing amounts to an assurance that if death cannot be staved off, lives nevertheless may be "saved" another way. French philosopher Gabriel Marcel offered an account that is revealing and relevant to the descriptions offered in so much testimony about AIDS.[38] In his analysis, testimony is always subjective, bearing on an event that is unique and irrevocable: testimony always comes after. If events or lives could be reconstructed, testimony would be superfluous. But events and lives are lost, and testimony is the only way in which it is possible to preserve a sense of the worth and merit of persons: "To witness is to act as guarantor."

Thus construed, testimony is even morally obligatory inasmuch as it is an essential part of our relationships with one another, as much as honesty or fidelity. Grief and mourning are not therefore only psychological states serving cathartic resolution of grief or anguish. The open affirmation and willingness to face disbelief which define testimony are part of morality itself. Testimony is thus a judgment of worth, an estimate of loss, an acknowledgment of limitations, and for those who remain behind an opportunity for intimacy.[39] Testimony about the dead is not driven by a desire to overcome death but to prevent it from eroding the meaningfulness of life. Testimony, not death, is the last word.

The worth of writing and speaking in protest or lament is not to be undervalued; it is something, after all, other than tears writ large. It is certainly true that reading about AIDS to delight in the suffering of one's moral enemies would be ghoulish, yet it would be worse, by several orders of magnitude, if there were no writing at all about the epidemic

or the dead. The narratives about the dead with AIDS cannot by themselves generate lab space or produce educational programs, but they have
their place in the order of human needs. It is not surprising that these
narratives typically focus on the unique role the PWA held in the narrator's life (as son, friend, lover, husband) and those qualities that did
not deserve the end to which they came. This is why those narratives
which try to summarize a person by demographics of race, occupation,
and residence fail to be morally interesting or convincing. A testimony
is more than demographics. Neither does testimony attempt to substitute words for persons; that would be mere fetishism. Testimony is
witness before an indifferent world about the worth and merit of persons.
And thus one writes for a world unconvinced that someone was here and
that, death notwithstanding, a presence remains.

Personal names loom large in AIDS testimony because we understand
names as symbols of persons, not as summaries. The effort in AIDS
testimony to ensure that names endure, names like Peter VonLehn,
Roger Horwitz, and Eddie Mickler, can also be seen in those memorials
that typically insist on the primacy of names. All of these shun the horror
of mass graves. In the years following World War II the Imperial War
Graves Commission listed in page after page of the seven volumes of the
Civilian War Dead in the United Kingdom 1939–1945 the names of
civilians killed in the course of the war, many of whom were killed by
bombs falling on their homes. Inside the west door of Westminster
Abbey in London one of these volumes is always open to display the
names of some of those who died: "George Alfred Yeomans. Age 46;
of 10 Troutbeck Road. Husband of Laura Rose Yeomans. 2 August
1944 at 10 Troutbeck Road," or "Beryl June Yeomans. Age 15; of 10
Troutbeck Road. Daughter of George Alfred Yeomans. 2 August 1944
at 10 Troutbeck Road." Like this register of persons, the Vietnam
Memorial in Washington is finally remarkable not because of its materials, form, or design but because it found room for the name of every
person who died during that divisive conflict and is thus a reminder that
such testimonials are not finally about art but about persons.

Literary critic Jeff Nunokawa has pointed out that there is a deep
cultural presumption associating male homosexuality with death as a
foreordained extinction.[40] A cultural tradition which defines death as an
essential attribute of gay men, of course, places unique demands on
writers who reject that damning linkage. Some memorialists so want to
distance their dead from the tradition of "deadly" homosexuality that
they take pains, even on panels in the Names Project, to state the route

of infection so that the deceased is not stigmatized with homosexuality and its imagined evils. This kind of cemeterial apartheid, of course, extends the cultural presumption that some people with AIDS are and some are not "innocent" victims: there are those who develop AIDS following a blood transfusion, artificial insemination, or robust hetero-sexual promiscuity, as in the case of Magic Johnson, and then there are gay men.

It is a challenge to memorialize men who are generally supposed to be responsible for their own death. It is also difficult to memorialize gay men without invoking and reinforcing the view that homosexuality leads ineluctably to death, especially when other views of the lives of gay men are pervasively and systematically absent from the media of entertain-ment and education. Many of the writers discussed here have met this challenge inasmuch as they create what Nunokawa has called alternative obituaries.[41] While some experiences have been fictionalized, first-per-son narratives and obituaries are the primary venue for writing about those who have died with AIDS. This writing remains primarily the province of gay authors and readers, if only because gay authors and readers find obstacles in venues outside their control. Some newspapers, for example, will not list gay lovers in obituaries, even if the relationship had existed for years, even if the biological family had long since been geographically and emotionally absent.[42] Gay newspapers, by contrast, routinely name surviving partners and often use the word "lover" in place of the usage preferred by some mainstream papers, "companion." They will often mention the number of years the men spent together and, along with blood relatives, may also cite the friends who from day to day became a gay man's family. By themselves, of course, testimonials written for gay men will not rectify larger cultural views that gay identity is necessarily doomed, but they do offer gay men the opportunity to speak with their own voice about the meaning, their meaning of their lives and death.

While struggle about public representations of gay men continues even in regard to their obituaries, it is characteristic nevertheless of all obituaries, regardless of their policies about survivors, to find what kind word there is to say of the dead, whether he or she is the chairman of a university academic department, a Roman Catholic priest, a bartender, or a librarian. As a matter of preserving the meaning of lives, testimony in fiction, eulogy, and monument is a moral act. It is the moral heart of writing about the epidemic. It is the essence of the deeply personal Names Project. Testimony is an essential part of any moral analysis of the epidemic. It is an important way by which to challenge the public mythology about promiscuous, fast-track, unloving gay men. The grief of the epidemic and the incentive to memorialize are no mere biological reflexes; they are an assertion against the leveling effect of death that persons are not replaceable, that death does not nullify presence. They can also be important embodiments of moral wisdom and vehicles of social criticism.

In *Borrowed Time* the metaphor Monette invokes to represent the experience of AIDS is that of living on the moon. But it is clear that Monette does not intend the moon as the faithful, consoling light of the night sky, the Roman patroness of the hunt. He invokes the moon as a barren and lifeless expanse inhospitable to human hope and love.[43] Only those who know the epidemic firsthand can know what this desolation is like, Monette says; those who live in the lush expanse of good health cannot appreciate the hopes and fears AIDS brings, cannot appreciate the rarity of abundant health. It is no wonder then that Monette finally blurts out to a friend: "I'm not going to be around long myself, and I don't want to talk to people without AIDS anymore."[44]

But in their writings Monette and all the others mentioned here *do* talk to people without AIDS. Indeed, they will be talking to people with and without AIDS as long as their writing endures. They do so because the failure to testify would amount to betrayal, would be continuous in meaning with the absurdity of the epidemic. The personal narratives of those dead and dying of AIDS may have ambitions in regard to social reformation and medical advance, but they all begin as the story of an individual life, an individual person. This kind of narrative is nothing so much as a will to preserve in ink and paper the virtues of persons that are lost in the more evanescent medium of flesh. It is what way there is to resist the absurdity of suffering and death. To be sure, memorial testimony is not the only form of discourse required to speak against the absurdities of suffering and death, especially to the extent the epidemic is abetted by political and social cowardice and hypocrisy, but it is a necessary voice and one that has moral import even where it reveals only the homely truths that we deserve better than we get, that we mourn more than the world can know, that we are each other's only refuge.

PART TWO

HIV Testing

4

Celebrities and AIDS

A 1992 letter to the editor of the *New England Journal of Medicine* calls attention to the increase in HIV tests at an anonymous test site in Orange County, California, following a celebrity's public disclosure of an HIV-related death, infection, or illness.[1] The authors even graph the occurrence of HIV testing at that site, noting the highest occurrences of HIV testing at the time of Liberace's and Rock Hudson's deaths and after announcements of HIV infection or illness by California property tax opponent Paul Gann, basketball star Earvin "Magic" Johnson, and tennis champion Arthur Ashe. Celebrities with AIDS have formed an integral part of the public history of the HIV epidemic in the United States. The fame some people already knew was given new dimensions by their deaths with AIDS: French philosopher Michel Foucault in 1984, U.S. House Representative Stuart McKinney in 1987,[2] and "Psycho" star Anthony Perkins in 1992[3] among them. AIDS has even conferred on some celebrity they would not otherwise have had: Ryan White, an Indiana boy barred from his local school;[4] Fabian Bridges, a transient hustler who prompted national debate about the responsibility and limits of public health authority;[5] Kimberly Bergalis, a Florida college student who incurred an HIV infection at the hands of her dentist; Ali Gertz, a heterosexual woman who was infected during a single sexual encounter with a bisexual man;[6] and even Belinda Mason, a self-described Tupperware housewife from Kentucky who served for a time until her death on the National Commission on AIDS.[7]

The authors of the *New England Journal* letter advance the view that celebrities should be enlisted in efforts to control AIDS, at a minimum by going public with their diagnoses. The question of celebrity disclosure and its power to help control the epidemic is worth considering for what it suggests about efforts necessary to control AIDS, especially the role of HIV testing. Despite its association with increased HIV testing at an anonymous test center, there are many reasons to think that celebrity disclosure is an inappropriate cornerstone on which to build an approach to control the HIV epidemic in the United States. Not only does reliance on celebrity disclosure presume certain questionable conclusions about HIV testing and the nature of the patient-physician relationship but advocacy of celebrity disclosure as important to the control of the epidemic reveals that HIV has failed to be understood as the permanently and inexorably important health risk it is. Celebrity disclosures about their diagnoses, moreover, have contained mixed messages about the meaning of AIDS, messages that constrain the ability to confront AIDS openly and effectively.

The Uses of Fame in an Epidemic

The four authors of the *New England Journal* letter write that "although there can be no question that unauthorized disclosure of HIV infection or the onset of AIDS in well-known figures is an invasion of personal privacy, such disclosures have an impressive effect on public health. In Orange County, California, such disclosures have been followed by sustained increases in the use of anonymous ('alternative test site') HIV-antibody testing." The benefit of voluntary disclosure about an HIV-related condition by famous people is said to serve the instrumental good of unifying an otherwise culturally partitioned society:

In a society as fragmented along lines of race, culture, age, and socioeconomic class as the United States, the recognition and love of pop-culture celebrities are rare unifying features that represent an opportunity to overcome barriers to communication. The more frequently members of America's royal family choose to alarm and motivate the public about AIDS through personal disclosure, the more successful will be our national effort to control this disease. Disclosure by celebrities may also serve to promote nondiscrimination against those with the HIV infection.

While it is important to recognize, as this letter does, the importance of efforts to "control this disease" and to "promote nondiscrimination," the way this control is sought suffers from conceptual and moral difficulties that overwhelm the benefit of celebrity involvement with AIDS. First of all, the language used by the letter shows that the authors apparently believe that alarm is the best way to alert the public to the dangers of AIDS and that celebrity disclosure is an unparalleled opportunity for such alarm. But is alarming the public about AIDS the best strategy for the control of the disease? Is alarming people about AIDS the best strategy for *educating* people about the syndrome, its means of infection, its consequences, or techniques for its avoidance? Alarming people may have entirely the opposite effect, for it may provoke entirely inappropriate individual and social responses to the epidemic, ranging from personal denial of risk to authoritarian civic measures inspired by fear and homophobia. Certain reports have made clear that some Americans are prepared to tolerate discrimination against PWAs[8] and some health professionals recognize no professional obligation to care for patients with AIDS.[9] Moreover, in time an approach that presumes the utility of alarm may soon find an audience deadened to messages about the importance of HIV risk avoidance. A condition of permanent alarm is almost a contradiction in terms. Enough alarms have already been sounded about AIDS in the last decade—from pamphlets addressed to American households by the U.S. Surgeon General to tabloid and news magazine headlines galore—that it is a wonder there are any ways left to vary the message about the evils of AIDS. Thus celebrity-provoked, panicked responses to AIDS do not seem capable of promoting the sustained efforts necessary to reach people with messages and assistance that can translate fear of AIDS into effective ways of avoiding HIV infection across the entirety of one's life. The choice of the word "alarm" may have been unfortunate, but that four individuals authored the letter suggests that the wording was deliberate. No one disagrees that AIDS should be approached as a gravely important personal and social issue, but it remains unproven that alarm of the public by its vaunted public figures is the best way to direct and sustain educational efforts about HIV risk avoidance.

The authors of this *New England Journal of Medicine* letter assume that greater testing affords more opportunity to control AIDS than does less testing. Nothing in the data offered in their letter, however, supports such a contention. There is nothing in their graphed representation of the use of the alternative HIV test site that shows that increased HIV testing affords more control over the epidemic just because testing is more frequent (see figure 1). For example, in November 1991, following

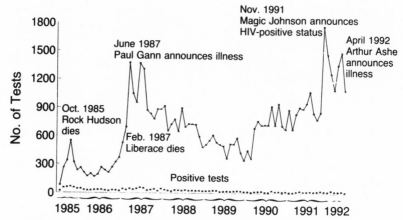

1. This graph plots the use of an anonymous HIV test site in Orange County, California, from July 1985 through May 1992. Reprinted, by permission, from *New England Journal of Medicine* 327 (1992): 1389.

Magic Johnson's disclosure of his HIV infection, the alternative HIV test site in Orange County reported about 1,800 HIV tests, the highest number of tests ever performed there. And yet the number of HIV infections discovered through such testing was equal to or even sometimes less than the number of infections discovered when testing rates were at their lowest, when there was no correlated HIV disclosure by a celebrity. There is nothing in the data to suggest that more persons discovered an HIV infection at this test site because they were moved to seek testing subsequent to a celebrity disclosure than if they had come at times unconnected with celebrity disclosure, than if they had come for reasons associated with recognition of personal HIV risk behavior or symptomatology.

What is striking about the HIV test rates reported in this letter is not only how much testing increases following a celebrity disclosure but how infrequently such panic-motivated testing leads to increased discovery of HIV infection. Indeed, in the wake of a celebrity disclosure, the percentage of tests that led to an identified infection *decreased* dramatically. Testing increased between Rock Hudson's death and Magic Johnson's announcement of his HIV infection by about 200 percent, yet there was virtually no increase in the number of HIV infections detected by such testing. We may see such testing therefore not as a triumph of "AIDS awareness" but as a failure of the public to know when HIV testing is appropriate. That failure may be all the more significant since six years of AIDS educational efforts transpired between Hudson's death and Johnson's announcement. The rush to testing may therefore suggest that the public does not understand how HIV is contracted or what its symptoms are.

An underlying assumption in this letter also bears consideration: that testing is an unqualified good. Testing may be an equivocal good indeed if it is filling public educational and psychological needs that are otherwise inadequately met. That so many people can be panicked into unnecessary tests shows that the rush to testing following a celebrity disclosure has less to do with personal risk of HIV infection than with larger social fears about the incidence and prevalence of AIDS or maybe, more accurately, the media incidence and the media prevalence of AIDS. If people seek an HIV test because they hear reports that a well-known property tax reformer or sports figure has AIDS, we begin to wonder if people believe HIV can be transmitted through the exchange of ink and electricity, through *media fluids*. News about celebrities with AIDS thus assumes for some the status of risk factor for HIV infection, alongside unsafe sex and dirty needle use.

Identification of HIV infection is unquestionably an important diagnostic event for the management of personal illness. Yet the negative results of the many tests reported in the *New England Journal* letter indicate that the general public is not necessarily at personal risk of HIV infection but that people are afraid that AIDS may be seeping out of the risk groups in which it was epidemiologically and culturally "contained." Testing is one way to assure members of a nervous public that they are not infected, that there is still distance between them and the epidemic. Media announcements by celebrities seem to prompt these people to suspect that—for reasons utterly beyond their control or knowledge—they too are infected. Thus construed, the increased use of HIV testing reveals a cultural panic at the perceived collapse of the moral and conceptual barriers people have erected between themselves and HIV.

HIV Diagnosis and Patient-Physician Relations

The *New England Journal of Medicine* authors also emphasize the responsibility of physicians to promote disclosure by celebrities of any HIV-related condition: "In weighing the good of the many against that of individuals—in this case, patients—physicians should actively but supportively encourage HIV-positive celebrities to publicly disclose their status. And though the individual prerogative to decline disclosure must be respected, the physician's responsibility as protector of the public health should not be easily dismissed." Such counsel is questionable on a number of grounds. The authors stipulate that the good of the many must be weighed against the good of the individual patients. But framing the justification this way is to prove too much: What individual interest is there that could prove inviolable when weighed against the hypothetical good of the many, that is, of *all others*? The very approach here—that the good of the many is decisive—structures the issue prejudicially against individuals' interests. On such an approach the individual then bears the burden of proof as to why his or her interests should be respected as against the greater—by definition—interests of the general public. Such a view genuinely risks collapsing the private into the public, extinguishing the lines between personal and social interests because an individual could have no responsibilities or rights other than those serving the general good. Such blurring of private and public has occurred before in the epidemic, of course, but the effect is particularly serious here since it challenges a medical tradition that has typically put the patient's interests at the center of all decision-making. If it becomes the physician's responsibility to balance both the interests of the patient and of the many at the same time, the physician will of necessity approach patients with the potential for divided loyalty or with the potential for seeing patients as natural resources to be used in campaigns toward whatever social goals that physician might identify as important.

It is also unclear why the authors deem the physician as primarily responsible for cultivating celebrity support in the fight against AIDS. True, physicians will have knowledge of individual celebrity's diagnoses, but why should they any more than attorneys or ministers have the responsibility for actively recruiting individuals into campaigns against AIDS? In other words, it is unclear why—just because he or she has access to diagnostic information—it falls to the physician as a matter of professional obligation (and the letter uses the obligatory language of "should") to find ways to put celebrities before news conferences. Would a physician be failing in any aspect of his or her individual responsibility *to a patient* if he or she were *never* to urge a celebrity patient to go public with a diagnosis? The central question raised by the letter is whether physicians ought to recruit their patients into involvements that the physicians have identified as important, involvements that are extraneous to the purposes for which a person—celebrity or not—seeks a physician. Even if the discovery of HIV infections had increased after celebrity disclosures, it is hard to see why physicians have any more duty in regard to the social goal of decreasing HIV infection than to decreasing syphilis or other illnesses or disabilities. One might respond that physicians should enlist all patients into efforts in which their celebrity might help a worthwhile social cause, but such a response—while diminishing concerns about selective use of patients—would be even further susceptible to questions about the erosion of distinctions between private and public, between the personal and the social. Such a response would strain mightily the presumption of confidentiality in health-care relations.[10]

Any question of the recruitment of patients for important social goals goes to the heart of the patient-physician relationship. In these days it is naive to suggest that there can be a single generally valid model for all health-care relationships, especially given the way the delivery of health care is fractured by a variety of institutions and health professionals. On the contrary, there are many legitimate forms of interaction shaped by the context in which patients and physicians encounter one another. There are even reasons to see some such relationships as having adversarial components.[11] Nonetheless, recruiting celebrities to disclose HIV-related conditions seems fairly inappropriate on most models of physician-patient encounters, unless it is granted that physicians may recruit patients for whatever other purposes they wish. Of course, patients are in fact frequently recruited into pharmaceutical and surgical trials, for example, in ways that do not necessarily imply the undivided loyalty of physicians. But there is a crucial difference here: most persons in such trials are enrolled because they are the only persons whose condition affords the possibility of testing drugs and surgical techniques. But it has not been demonstrated that widespread efforts to educate against HIV infection could not proceed, with success and without alarm, without the efforts of individual celebrities as urged in the *New England Journal* letter.

The authors do acknowledge that a patient's decision not to disclose an HIV infection should be respected, but the last sentence of the letter asserts a moral authority that functions by its tone and placement to diminish the standing of the patient in this regard: "And though the individual prerogative to decline disclosure must be respected, the physician's responsibility as protector of the public health should not be easily dismissed." While the authors do use the language of obligation ("must") in limiting the physician's right to seek disclosure, they also impute to physicians a moral grandeur that functionally diminishes the standing of a patient who would not willingly collaborate with a "pro-tector of the public health." The connotative force of such language conjures the physician as mediating a conflict between an individual and the public health as a whole. (It is interesting that only one of the four authors of the letter has an M.D. degree.) On such a scale a celebrity's unwillingness to disclose an AIDS diagnosis—as in the case of Arthur Ashe's initial reluctance—appears if not outright selfishness then at least as a significant waste of significant resources.[12] Certainly, celebrities like Ryan White[13] and Magic Johnson[14] have made it easier for people to talk about and take up AIDS as the important issue that it is, but there is nothing in the relationship of physician to patient that requires efforts to enlist them in the fight against AIDS, especially if those efforts cast celebrity patients into compromises with their own conscience and into morally suspect altruism.

If the control of AIDS depends on alarms sounded by celebrity disclosure and if the patient-physician relationship can be structured by the social needs of the day, then the battle against the epidemic is probably already lost. If people are willing to submit to HIV testing primarily because a celebrity whom they recognize acknowledges an HIV-related diagnosis, then anti-AIDS efforts stand indicted of grave social and educational failings despite half a generation's work. The *New England Journal* letter authors say that celebrity disclosure has "an impressive effect on the public health." Yet neither the prevention of new HIV infection nor the decrease in discriminatory attitudes toward people with AIDS can be demonstrated as an effect of celebrity disclo-sure; moreover, if the goal of celebrity disclosure is "alarm," how can we expect more tolerance and humanity? Certainly, no reform of the health-care system can result from such an approach, and such a panicked response cannot advance individual understanding of the risk of HIV infection, promote techniques for avoidance of such risk, or effect the incidence or prevalence of HIV disease. Despite all the various celebrity disclosures that have taken place during the epidemic, still many people fail to take measures to protect themselves from HIV risk.[15]

Celebrity AIDS

Celebrities do have a number of important functions to play in response to the epidemic. Some celebrities have become involved with AIDS education, Whoopi Goldberg, for example, and many celebrities now wear a looped red ribbon at highly visible events like the Emmy and Oscar presentations as a "symbol of AIDS awareness." Elizabeth Taylor was instrumental in founding the American Foundation for AIDS Research and has inaugurated another AIDS agency.[16] Arthur Ashe also created and sought funding for an organization of his own.[17] Celebrities can help raise money for research and treatment through the organizations they create or support, and they elicit media attention when present at AIDS benefits and governmental hearings. They can also help individuals identify with the epidemic by legitimating the epidemic as an object of concern. The involvement of such individuals as author Larry Kramer[18] in anti-AIDS efforts can also strengthen personal and governmental commitment to the control of the epidemic. Insofar as such activism involves unambiguously straight persons, celebrity presence can help some people put aside the notion that only "homosexuals" and drug-users have a vested interest in AIDS. Celebrities can help people set aside the notion that they will be suspected of immorality or complicity with immorality by evincing any interest whatsoever in AIDS. That public figures have to help counter such attitudes is an indictment of American cultural and social taboos that interfere with thorough and effective anti-HIV education insofar as such efforts reveal the barriers that prejudicially divide this democratic society.

While there are benefits of celebrity involvement in fighting AIDS, it would be a mistake to put celebrities at the cornerstone of that fight and not only because celebrity disclosure does not by itself educate about effective HIV risk avoidance. This "disclosure" may also conceal as much as it reveals. Doctors and family members who announced Foucault's death for example made no mention of AIDS. One French historian has labeled Foucault's silence about his AIDS the silence of shame about his sexuality.[19] Rock Hudson, in the statement publicly acknowledging his AIDS (he did not even make the statement himself, leaving it to another to face the cameras), denied knowledge of how he contracted an HIV infection. In fact, he had initially denied that he had AIDS and had even lied to his lover when that man directly asked whether Hudson had AIDS. (A court subsequently held that Hudson's lies justified awarding a considerable portion of Hudson's estate to his lover, Marc Christian.[20]) Designer Perry Ellis's death was attributed technically and correctly to encephalitis, leaving it to the public at large to connect that diagnosis to the CDC definition of AIDS. The HIV infection that caused the death of Congressman Stuart McKinney was attributed by his physicians to transfusions "as the most logical source." Shortly afterward, however, a male lover appeared who declared the congressman had sexual relations with men. Ironically, his physicians had noted that McKinney "wanted the cause of his death known after he passed away, in hopes that this information might help others to deal with what is becoming a national crisis."[21] Similarly, newscaster Max Robinson denied the nature of his illness prior to his 1988 death with AIDS, although according to statements made by friends after his death, he wanted his death to emphasize the need for AIDS awareness among blacks.[22] Actor Robert Reed's 1992 death with HIV-related conditions was initially covered up until his death certificate became public.[23] Tennis champion and author Arthur Ashe did finally disclose his illness but only to preempt a national paper from breaking the story in a sensationalizing way. Randy Shilts, the author of one of the most important volumes about the beginnings of the AIDS epidemic and one of the very few nationally known and openly gay journalists in this country, also disclosed his AIDS diagnosis only in order to stave off an involuntary "outing" in the media.[24] Despite widespread and well-placed rumors, Rudolph Nureyev never openly acknowledged a diagnosis of AIDS; after his 1993 death his physician initially disclosed only that the famous ballet dancer had died of cardiac complications following a grievous disease.[25]

One public disclosure of a celebrity's HIV diagnosis—one not cited in the *New England Journal* letter—came as a surprise even to him. According to statements by his wife, Anthony Perkins first learned *through the tabloids* that he had an HIV infection.[26] Having been treated at a hospital for a condition unrelated to AIDS, Perkins's blood was apparently tested for HIV without his knowledge and the report of an infection was sold to a tabloid that put the story on its front page. Perkins subsequently sought confirmation of his diagnosis but spoke publicly about his condition through a letter released only after his death. Even then full disclosure was not forthcoming. When asked if she knew how Perkins had contracted an HIV infection, his wife said, "No. We really don't know. It's not worth it."[27] Before him, actor Brad Davis released information about his disease only after his death, noting that a public disclosure of HIV would have ruined his career.[28] Others have never acknowledged their AIDS. Only an ordered autopsy, for example, confirmed AIDS as the cause of Liberace's death.[29]

Many of these celebrity "disclosures" are evidence of the social stigmatization of gay sex and drug use. They reveal what may and may not be spoken about openly, what does and does not damage a dead man's reputation. Apparently implications of homosexuality and drug use are greater threats to professional survival than any other allegation. The silence embedded in such "disclosures" may in fact offset any benefits of disclosure, for such silence reinforces cultural barriers to open and frank discussion of HIV risk, homoeroticism, and drug use. Celebrity disclosure by itself clearly does not ensure that the right messages are being delivered simply because the diagnoses of celebrities are involved. Douglas Crimp, for example, has noted that Magic Johnson's appearance on the "Arsenio Hall Show" the day following his public disclosure of HIV infection recapitulated a number of linguistic and conceptual forms of homophobia and misogyny. After Johnson told Arsenio, "I'm far from being homosexual," the audience thundered its approval, suggesting that an HIV infection notwithstanding Johnson had committed only venial sins and not transgressed the standards of public morality by violating heterosexual norms. Crimp also rightly noted the misogyny in Johnson's declarations about the circumstances of his HIV infection in which he portrayed women as sexual predators and himself as their victim.[30] These kinds of disclosures and discussions are ambiguous in their capacity for AIDS education. In Johnson's case his particular disavowal of homosexuality reaffirmed the legitimacy of homophobia and implicitly reaffirmed the assumption that it is gay sex and not AIDS that is the real public enemy. In effect, rather than serving as vehicles of public education, many disclosures and denials about AIDS have functioned instead as alibis against accusations of gay sex and drug use.

The benefits of celebrity disclosure should not be ignored, however. Magic Johnson's efforts subsequent to his disclose of HIV infection—participation in the U.S. Olympic basketball team, public advocacy of AIDS education, and even his resignation in protest from the National Commission on AIDS because its counsel was going unheeded by government—offer some important counterexamples to the public mythology of life devastated by HIV infection. Johnson also prepared a practical guide on how to avoid HIV risk (though the direct anatomical language in that book caused some major book retailers to decline stocking it).[31] Before his death Arthur Ashe also took up AIDS as a cause important to him and the nation. He wrote, lectured, and appeared on behalf of various anti-AIDS causes.[32] But these two individuals are the exceptions rather than the rule when it comes to celebrities with HIV-related conditions who have committed themselves to anti-AIDS efforts.

Arthur Ashe did urge more celebrities and entertainers to enlist in the fight against AIDS because of the impression such persons make on impressionable eighteen-year-olds.[33] He said he thought celebrities could reach eighteen-year-olds in ways that other HIV educators could not. Certainly, one clear benefit of celebrity involvement is that people may begin to talk more openly about AIDS and display more compassion for PWAs; disclosures make it harder for the public to maintain the kind of malice and prejudice possible when AIDS "victims" remain an unidentified, invisible population rather than public figures for whom one has admiration.

HIV Testing and Celebrity Disclosure

Celebrities can indeed draw attention to AIDS, but insofar as their declarations are framed by homophobic and other prejudicial attitudes, they also divert attention as well. Given that celebrity disclosures can only be random and occasional, public health efforts should not rely on them to carry an important part of HIV educational efforts. Indeed, reliance on celebrities might work against AIDS education in an ironic way. To the extent that the "general public" does not see itself involved in gay sex or needle-sharing, it sees AIDS as a distant risk significant only to "others." In the same way, if people do not perceive themselves living the opulent life of celebrities, they can merely understand celebrities as yet another risk group without educational significance for their own sex and drug-using lives.

If all this seems like so much sniping in response to one letter to a medical journal, let me say on the contrary that the letter captures certain cultural assumptions that affirm an uncritical blessing of widespread HIV testing and that situate control of the epidemic in ad hoc reactions to public events. The letter's appearance as the lead feature of the correspondence section in one of the world's foremost medical journals situates it as an important cultural artifact. It would have been a more telling letter, however, had it reported conclusions contrary to those it offered. Had the letter reported that celebrities' disclosures had no effect on use of anonymous HIV test sites, we might have evidence that people better understand the nature of HIV risk and symptoms and seek testing only as individually appropriate. As it is, testing centers draw people in merely because of celebrity disclosures.

Should celebrities wish to come forward for reasons of their own—and Arthur Ashe was right that more celebrity involvement is welcome—one hopes that their disclosures will neither panic the public nor be framed in ways that implicitly incriminate gay men and drug-users as responsible for the epidemic. Celebrity efforts—indeed all educational efforts—should avoid denials that AIDS is a gay disease if such denials imply that AIDS would be a less pressing health concern if it affected only gay men or that AIDS is important only to the extent that it spreads beyond gay men. One hopes too that such disclosures may join but not displace the many and on-going community efforts that are already underway. To pretend that the fight against AIDS must begin *ab initio* at each celebrity diagnosis would wrongly obscure the heroic efforts already initiated and maintained without the luster of celebrity support. In the final analysis it is not the celebrity but the obscure person who ought to be the focus of efforts against AIDS, and it is with every such person that a physician might properly begin efforts to protect the "public health," not by urging disclosure of HIV infections but by counseling the uninfected and the unfamous on how to stay that way.

5

The Angry Death
of Kimberly Bergalis

Among celebrities with AIDS, Kimberly Bergalis has received a great deal of attention from the United States media. She thus belongs alongside filmstar Rock Hudson,[1] Ryan White, basketball player Magic Johnson,[2] and tennis player Arthur Ashe, whose life stories have constituted a significant part of the public narrative of AIDS in the United States. Bergalis was the Florida college student whose AIDS was traced by the CDC to HIV infection from her dentist in 1987.[3] The CDC subsequently identified other persons whose AIDS was also traceable to infection in the course of treatment by that same dentist. Other cases of AIDS in patients had, of course, already been linked to health-care settings, most notably through blood transfusions but also through artificial inseminations and organ transplantation. Certain accidental HIV exposures of health-care workers, primarily through needle-stick injuries, have also led to their infection and subsequent sickness and death.[4] Bergalis, however, was the first person whose AIDS was linked to HIV infection in the course of treatment that did not involve those other means of infection. That her infection came at the hands of her dentist made Bergalis's infection one of the most prominent occurrences of AIDS in the United States. That the specific means of her infection was never identified made her infection a focus of public alarm and policy analysis. Bergalis was also by all accounts among the publicly angriest persons to have AIDS. After her diagnosis, Bergalis did not privately rail against the dying of the light, she railed against those she thought responsible for her illness and eventual death, and she called on government officials and the health professions to test health-care workers for HIV. Joining a host of voices raised about the importance of responding to the epidemic, Bergalis and her family championed the cause of HIV testing. Are there lessons from her anger that ought to be heeded in formulating AIDS public policy, especially in regard to testing health-care workers for HIV?

Testing Health-Care Workers for HIV

Bergalis's ordeal began in 1989 when her mother noticed her declining health and she was subsequently diagnosed with AIDS. Because Bergalis appeared to have none of the usual risk factors for HIV infection, her illness was of some epidemiological interest. DNA tests by the CDC linked her HIV infection to her dentist, though the CDC failed to identify any specific incident or mechanism that permitted this kind of dentist-to-patient infection.[5] Bergalis's dentist, David Acer, had apparently known for a number of years that he had an HIV infection, but he had evidently not told any clients about his condition. He thereby preempted any choice on their part whether to continue receiving dental care from him.[6] Bergalis and others saw such silence as an arrogation of their privilege to choose the risks to which they would voluntarily submit. Apart from the issue of disclosure to patients, Bergalis and her family also frequently expressed anger that there was no policy barrier to practice by dentists and other health-care workers with HIV-related conditions. In a letter to Florida health officials Bergalis once wrote: "I blame Dr. Acer and every single one of you bastards. Anyone who knew Dr. Acer was infected and had full-blown AIDS and stood by not doing a damn thing about it. You are all just as guilty as he was. You've ruined my life and my family's. If laws are not formed to provide protection, then my suffering and death was in vain."[7]

Bergalis's public ordeal culminated in October 1991 when in a highly debilitated condition she made a trip by train from her home in Florida to the nation's capital to offer personal testimony before a congressional committee. That hearing was convened to gather information about proposed federal legislation that would require HIV testing of all health-care workers, legislation that was in fact named in honor of Bergalis. Her trip was attended by news media all along the way, and there was considerable speculation about the impact her appearance itself would have since it was already known that she was in favor of such mandatory HIV testing. Dying with AIDS, the frail Bergalis was expected to make a commanding witness, testifying with all the authority of her ill health against the complacency of the federal government that endangered patients nationwide. In the end, however, she offered only a few, short sentences of testimony and did not specify what form she would like HIV protection in health-care relations to take. Instead she reasserted her innocence and without identifying exactly what should be done called on Congress to do *something:* "I did not do anything wrong, yet I am being made to suffer like this. My life has been taken away. Please enact legislation so that no other patient or health-care provider will have to go through the hell that I have."[8]

In one sense Bergalis helped advance the cause of AIDS education in the way the Indiana teenager Ryan White did before her as he and his mother fought AIDS discrimination. Because she represented a kind of person who, according to a certain moral view, should by all rights be worriless about the epidemic,[9] her illness made it possible and easier for others to talk about AIDS without having to worry about the homo-erotic and narcotic associations that have shrouded the epidemic in this country. By discussing AIDS through the "normalizing" filter of Kimberly Bergalis, people outside the putative risk groups of gay men, drug-using men and women, and their children could raise for themselves the question of possible HIV infection. Here, after all, was a young woman who got an HIV infection for no obvious morally punitive reason: perhaps such a person with AIDS could make clear for many people that the opposite of high risk is *low* risk, not no risk. And certainly her illness and death showed that HIV infection is possible in the health-care setting for other reasons than blood transfusions, needle-stick injuries, and artificial insemination. Not a "threatening" person either in appearance or behavior, Bergalis offered many people a way to identify with the harms of the epidemic and to appreciate its evils.

The interest of the American public in Bergalis's illness and death has a precedent in the media treatment of a small group of persons earlier featured on the cover of a national magazine. In 1985 *Life* proclaimed on its July cover: "NOW NO ONE IS SAFE FROM AIDS." The novelty that apparently justified that headline and its three-inch all capital red letters was that the persons featured in the accompanying article were outside the apparent risk groups for AIDS.[10] One subject was a heterosexual woman, one a heterosexual man, and the others all members of a Pennsylvania family, three of whom had AIDS.[11] There were allegedly no gay men in the article, no drug-users, no prostitutes. The text of "The New Victims"—which carried no byline—said that "the AIDS minorities are beginning to infect the heterosexual, drug-free majority."[12] The attraction of these people, like that of Bergalis, for the media was that they were stricken with AIDS even though they were ostensibly "outside" the groups mythically taken to define HIV risk. Moreover, someone *infected them* in ways unrelated to their personal failings.

In many ways the media narratives about Bergalis replayed the themes of this *Life* photoarticle. One way to gauge that the attention given to Bergalis belonged to her circumstances as a person outside a conventional risk group is to ask this question: Would there have been equivalent media attention had it been a gay man who contracted an HIV infection from this same dentist? Or would his AIDS have been invisible against the background of so many other tens of thousands of instances of "gay AIDS"? Would the story be something other than backpage newspaper filler even if he were believed in his claim that it was his dentist and not his sexual partners who was the occasion of infection? The kind of public attention given to Bergalis, for instance, was not—not even a fraction of it—directed to a gay police officer in California who acquired an HIV infection occupationally. In that case police officer Thomas Cady spent three years trying to convince his employers that his HIV infection was acquired as the result of blood splashes during the arrest of an HIV-infected suspect. It took the declaration of an administrative law judge to establish that his infection was occupationally acquired and that he was therefore eligible for health-care costs, disability pay, and possible retirement benefits.[13] Although Cady was infected for no immoral reasons (on the contrary, as a policeman on duty he was in fact supporting society's official moral order), his infection did not provoke the attention or worry that followed that of Kimberly Bergalis. One wonders therefore if the real issue driving media attention to Kimberly Bergalis wasn't the desire to reassure an anxious heterosexual public of its relative safety inasmuch as her kind of infection was rare and that AIDS was still not "leaking" out of its original risk groups.[14] As a gay man, Cady, by contrast, still belonged to a "risk group" and thus his unusual infection was subsumed into a cultural conflation of homoeroticism and AIDS and was therefore less worrisome by comparison.

It is worth noting too that Bergalis appeared before the nation as one of the relatively few publicly "respectable" females with AIDS at a time when most made the association of AIDS in women with prostitution, drug use, and other social disadvantages. Before her infection, Bergalis was a genial, unremarkable college student from a middle-class background and could be taken to represent certain idealized notions of womanly propriety and identity. She was therefore in a position to be easily portrayed as a "victim" of AIDS rather than, as many other less socially advantaged women with AIDS have been portrayed, its harbinger.[15]

Certainly Bergalis did draw national attention, and her misfortune set in motion much discussion about HIV and hepatitis safety in health-care settings. In response to her case, the U.S. Congress considered various legislative proposals regarding standards of health care and the CDC set about devising advisory recommendations for the practice of health-care professionals with HIV-related conditions.[16] But in another sense Bergalis and the train of events her illness set in motion may work against some AIDS educational and prevention efforts because of the moral assumptions underlying the blame she and her family assigned for her condition and because of her insistence on mandatory HIV testing. This is not to say that Bergalis did not suffer from her illness or to say that any health professional or legislator can be cavalier about the protection of patients in health care settings, but it is to say that Bergalis's views about the *meaning* of her infection and the *remedy* offered against such infection in fact depend on views that can work against effective protection from HIV infection.

Bergalis, for example, often angrily expressed the view that her illness could have been avoided had health professionals and government not been guilty of inaction, had they worked together to put in place a policy of mandatory HIV testing. Even if it was too late to save *her,* she argued, such a policy would be desirable for the future.[17] At the 1991 congressional hearing Bergalis's father, George, went further and plainly said of health-care workers with HIV: "Someone who has AIDS and continues to practice is nothing better than a murderer."[18] In his view, therefore, his daughter was murdered, and the failure by government and health organizations to act against health-care workers with HIV amounted to nothing less than complicity in murder.

Like many other PWAs before her, Bergalis and her family accused health professionals and government of deadly inaction. But the issue of inaction was understood differently by Bergalis: the message was not "Silence = Death" but "No Testing = Death." But is testing of health-care workers the answer to the problem posed by her infection? The advocacy of mandatory HIV testing suggests that an absolute barrier to accidental HIV infection in health-care relations is, first of all, possible. While HIV testing can be quite accurate, there will still be a range of false reports either wrongly identifying people as having HIV or failing to find them altogether. Moreover, such testing has no power to predict future infection in persons. To be effective, then, any policy of routine HIV testing would not only have to be universal and mandatory in order to assure that *all* workers were tested but it would also have to be continuous and carried on permanently in the future. Even thus implemented, given the fallibility and limitations of any testing technique and policy, it is unclear that all cases of HIV in health-care workers or patients would be "caught" by such a net. At present, for example, many teachers across the country go untested for tuberculosis even though such testing is required by states in which they work.

Other considerations also question the advisability of universal, mandatory, continuous HIV testing. For example, what should happen to those health-care workers discovered to have an HIV infection? Obviously, health-care workers would be immediately jeopardized in employment and possibly other important social and personal benefits. A durable minority of Americans is prepared to tolerate discrimination against people with AIDS.[19] To advocate a policy of HIV testing without also at the same time offering health-care workers protection from indefensible discrimination on the basis of their HIV infection is objectionably insensitive to the moral and civic interests of people with HIV. And it is worth mentioning again that the view that testing can protect the "general population" as noncombatants in the epidemic shares conceptual homologies of authority and control with views that HIV can and should be kept where it "belongs."[20] Richard D. Mohr, for example, has pointed out how such testing functions symbolically as a purification ritual to the detriment of gay men in service of the values of "heterosexual supremacy."[21]

Bergalis's characterization of her own blamelessness for AIDS recapitulates much of the moral phylogeny of AIDS in the United States. From the very beginning she claimed to have done nothing wrong. She asserted this view, for example, in a 1990 letter to Florida health officials: "Do I blame myself? I sure don't . . . I never used I.V. drugs, never slept with anyone, and never had a blood transfusion." Her father too thought of "morality" as a safeguard against AIDS: "Her sickness would have been easier to accept if she'd been a slut or a drug-user. But she had everything right."[22] From such a perspective Bergalis is thus defined as innocent in contrast with other people with AIDS whose "not-innocent actions" are thought to end almost inevitably in their infection. This dichotomy between innocent and culpable "victims" of AIDS has been a standard feature of public discourse since the onset of public moralizing about the epidemic.[23] If Bergalis's behavior was not immoral, so the argument would go, then it follows that *someone else's* immorality led to her condition. The passive language she chose to characterize her condition suggests that she saw herself as suffering at the hands of some malevolent agent: "and yet I am being made to suffer." The use of the present progressive tense also seems to suggest that the ongoing suffering could be lifted if only someone would help her. Other PWAs have rejected this posture of helplessness and taken it upon *themselves* to lift their burdens to the extent possible.

The dentist, David Acer, figures almost as a stock villain in this account: he was a bisexual with HIV, the kind of figure who by his hidden life forms the endangering bridge between gay men with HIV and otherwise "safe" heterosexual women. Acer even initially denied all possibility of infecting his clients.[24] The case thus reinforces the stereotypical villainy of the bisexual man who is also the predator of women, bringing to them the diseases exiled to homosexuality both by the rules of morality and epidemiology. Virtually assumed throughout this entire narrative is that the burdens of AIDS are malevolently imposed on "innocents" and that the control of AIDS will be found in a kind of moral quarantine enforced at the doors of doctors' offices.

After Bergalis's death certain reports began to surface that Acer had intentionally infected her and other patients.[25] An acquaintance of Acer's raised the possibility that the dentist had deliberately infected these patients in order to draw government attention to an epidemic that had not been taken seriously enough because the disease was killing only marginalized, socially rebuked men, women, and their children. The infection of people like Bergalis might thus hasten government action by involving sympathetic "victims." George Bergalis dismissed this possibility, however, believing the ill-substantiated reports to be part of a political campaign to diminish the merits of health-care worker testing. If Acer had intentionally rather than accidentally infected his patients, it would be unwarranted to institute a nationally coordinated plan against what was merely the work of a single malicious and now dead practitioner. The malevolent conspiracy implied in such speculations, however, reinforces the view of Acer as villain and his patients as victims, even if it does not support the necessity of government monitoring.

Representing Acer's patients as innocents falling prey to a predatory bisexual in the context of indifferent professional politics and slothful government policing suggests Bergalis's was a case of "immaculate infection," that is, one produced without sin. One of the remarkable features of her pathography is that her virginity ensured that her illness could only be interpreted as sexless. All the cultural connotations of children and sexlessness as innocent then come into play, and these connotations have the effect of reviving that unfortunate redundancy, the "innocent victim." Despite long-standing efforts on the part of PWAs to repudiate the confining connotations of the expression "AIDS victim,"[26] Bergalis played out her story of AIDS as exactly that, as a helpless and passive person. The word *victim* comes from the Latin *victima,* meaning a sacrificial animal, and this unfortunately seems to be how Bergalis represented herself, as dying for a cause: "If laws are not formed to provide protection, then my suffering and death was in vain."[27] She did not choose to call for health care for the socially disadvantaged with AIDS, and she did not call for more government funding for and scientific attention to AIDS.[28] Hers were angry calls for blanket protection that is in any case impossible to provide. And the anger did not end at her death. Immediately after Kimberly Bergalis's funeral, her mother stated that she would continue the fight for mandatory testing of all health-care workers,[29] and her family has continued to lobby on behalf of that testing.

Bergalis declined to join other PWAs who do not find in their experience of AIDS reasons for personal bitterness. By choosing bitterness, Bergalis rejected the view adopted by many PWAs that AIDS offers a chance to live fully on a daily basis.[30] Rather than undermining or sabotaging their lives, some PWAs have said that AIDS has transfigured and *enriched* their lives in ways that could not have otherwise happened. The view that a diagnosis of an HIV infection can transform a person's life for the better was expressed, for example, in a letter written to Ann Landers: "I now look at life in a totally different way. I no longer take for granted a sunny day, a beautiful flower or the small kindnesses of friends, I go out of my way to do favors for people. I am much more forthcoming with compliments and much less prone to make hurtful remarks. To put it bluntly, the virus has opened my eyes and made me a better person."[31] Thomas B. Stoddard, former director of the Lambda Legal Defense and Education Fund, put the matter this way: "I wouldn't wish this experience on anyone, but I find it absolutely fascinating. . . . It's rich, it's complex. It's filled with paradoxes. I'm very glad to be living this."[32] Clearly the notion of victim does not adequately describe the status of all PWAs, and bitterness need not be the only response to the disease.

Reliance on the notion of innocent victims of AIDS continues to perpetuate the view that except for knowing and culpable actions of certain persons there would be no HIV infection in persons beyond the "risk groups." Identifying herself by all the things she *had not* done, Bergalis suggested that HIV infection is permanently confined to gay men, drug-users, and their children, except for lapses of governmental quarantine in keeping those groups—whether they are health-care workers or not—away from all others. Her own analysis of her illness suggests that because she did not fall into those unhealthy groups, she should have remained permanently free of *any* risk. But these kinds of suggestions will not work as assumptions by which to approach HIV education and prevention. It is not clear that there is such a thing as a life free of HIV risk. It is not even clear that "risk groups" per se exist: only a minority of gay men, for example, have HIV-related conditions. It belongs to prejudice to believe that all gay men are and will remain at equivalent and inevitable risk of HIV infection and that all "others" are not at risk or at risk only through moral depredations inflicted on the unwilling. HIV risk belongs, in varying degrees, to *all* persons even if that risk is remote and unforeseeable. Such a recognition can begin to dismantle the belief that monitoring risk groups is what is essential for protection from HIV-related disease and to recast the matter as one of helping people protect themselves from HIV risks. It can also frame the agenda for the health professions as they try to image aggressive prophylactic measures that will protect patients and providers from one another.

The concepts of innocence and blame do not go very far in "explaining" the illnesses of people with AIDS. The lures of sex and drugs being what they are, it would be a harsh judgment to claim that people are not innocent because they are weak. Innocence and blamelessness come in forms other than virginity. It would be a harsh judgment to claim that people are not innocent because they are not sexual or narcotic virgins. Some teenagers, for example, contract an HIV infection despite all they know in general about the dangers of AIDS. Are they then *responsible* for their illness even though inexperienced in sexual and drug matters, inexperienced in gauging the long-term consequences of hasty choices? HIV infection still occurs in people who are fully aware of the risks of HIV infection, even in those who may themselves have lost friends and family members to AIDS. Perhaps the concept of innocence has no place in categorizing the classes of people with AIDS.[33] Instead of debating the merits of Bergalis's claim to innocence and her dentist's culpability, perhaps we would be better off if we instead evaluated the capacity of the health-care system to help PWAs. It proves a distraction from this latter task if we evaluate instead the moral fitness of people to benefit from the health-care system or their fitness for public sympathy.

If the life of Kimberly Bergalis had been a work of fiction, it is hard to see how it could have ended other than it did by reason of the characters at work there: a virgin girl, a protective family, a bisexual man, a disease "belonging" to homosexuality, an indolent legislature, and complacent health professions. What other story line could have drawn them together except some kind of conspiracy to effect her undoing and death? But her life was not a work of fiction; instead hers was a real life lost to AIDS, and that is lamentable enough in itself as the real and abiding misfortune that it is. There is no reason, though, to compound that sadness with bitterness, with angry recrimination when it is unclear that there is any policy that could have saved the first such "victim" as Bergalis. Debating the innocence of various people with AIDS will not help frame educational policies that will protect as many people as possible from AIDS, and mandatory HIV testing cannot deliver all the benefits attributed to it. It would bring dilemmas of its own.[34] To be sure, health-care institutions must find imaginative and aggressive ways to protect people in health-care services, but the question is whether imaginative and aggressive policies of prophylaxis might not achieve the same ends as a more stringent policy of HIV testing both of patients and workers. Measured against all treatments that might have caused HIV infection in a patient, the few cases caused by Dr. Acer appear vanishingly small not in individual importance but in their importance as an indictment of the safety of health-care practices in the age of AIDS.

Patient Protection and AIDS Activism

In the end Kimberly Bergalis's activism does not belong to that kind of constructive AIDS activism that calls for a rethinking of the categories through which we see and understand the epidemic. Neither was she an activist in the sense that she envisioned a redesign of the health-care system in order to make it more accessible and responsive to the care of all kinds of unhealthy and dying people. From the beginning to the end the impetus and moral of her story was fear. Her understanding of her illness and her projected institutional reforms suggested that there were hidden health-care workers whose reckless performance would infect persons entirely outside the risk groups to which HIV-related conditions have been morally and culturally confined. Save for those moral wretches and professional laggards, moral and "innocent" people would be free of HIV risk.

It is in fact important to find ways to free health-care relations from the fear of HIV infection—for both patient and provider—but routine, even mandatory HIV testing clearly cannot deliver what is being demanded in this regard. Bergalis's role as virgin and martyr dedicated to the cause of testing mystifies its limitations and creates an impossible standard of safety. Her dedication also mystifies a route of HIV infection that in absolute numbers and percentages is the least representative means of infection in the entire epidemic. Unwitting infection of patients is the most insignificant means of HIV infection in the history of the epidemic, and the total number of persons thus infected, *five,* pales by comparison with the over three hundred and thirty thousand cases of AIDS reported at this time from all other means of infection.[35] It would be wise if the kind of sustained attention given to Bergalis's life could be extended to those many, many more persons whose sexual and drug lives still put them in the way of HIV infection and whose human fallibility makes the development of effective therapies all the more pressing. In more than a coincidental way, sustained focus on the exceptional infection of Bergalis reinforces the very categories that have to be broken down before society recognizes that HIV disease belongs to humanity as its problem, not only to gay men and drug-users.

6

Health-Care Workers
with HIV

Do patients have the right to know whether their health-care providers have an HIV infection or have been diagnosed as having AIDS? The American Medical Association (AMA) asserted a limited right of exactly this kind in 1991, saying "The health of patients must always be the paramount concern of physicians." Until the uncertainty about transmission is resolved, the AMA held that HIV infected physicians should either abstain from performing invasive procedures which pose an identifiable risk of transmission or disclose their sero-positive status prior to performing a procedure and proceed only if there is informed consent.[1] While the AMA has subsequently retracted this standard of disclosure,[2] the desirability of such a broad requirement of disclosure given continued public concern about its safety is worth considering. I argue that patients do not have a generalized right to disclosure, not because patients do not have the right to protect themselves from unwanted risks but because HIV infection in health care does not ordinarily belong to the domain of disclosable risks because of its remote risk. Moreover, patients do not ordinarily have the duty to discern all risks to which they might be subjected in receiving health care. Even if patients are worried about HIV infection at the hands of their health-care practitioners, other measures than disclosure by those practitioners permit avoidance of the risk of HIV infection. Additionally, a patient's interest in knowing about an HIV/AIDS diagnosis in a health worker does not ordinarily have sufficient moral force by itself to justify involuntary disclosure when weighed against the interests a health worker may have in keeping such information private. In the course of this discussion I will not be considering all forms of HIV infection which may occur in health-care settings but only those involving infection by a health worker through such treatment as dental work or surgery. Though other means of HIV infection are important in their own right, I will not here take up the issue of HIV infection through the use of, for example, infected medical products, artificial insemination, or transplanted tissues.

HIV Infection and Health-Care Workers

As of October 1993 eleven health-care workers have been identified by the CDC as having been accidentally infected with HIV in the course of providing health care.[3] This reported number reflects only persons whose clinical condition meets the defining criteria of AIDS. There are other health workers, as many as eighty-two in the fall of 1992, whose asymptomatic HIV infection may have been occupationally, accidentally acquired.[4] The possibility of such infection led in the first instance to widespread discussion about the desirability and even perhaps the moral obligation to test all patients as they entered health-care settings, in order to allow health workers to exercise exposure-avoidance measures in the care of infected patients.[5] A parallel concern for patient protection raises the question of testing health workers. The concern I wish to address here is the patient's moral entitlement to knowledge of a health worker's HIV status. Does a patient have the right to seek and expect disclosure from any or all of his or her health workers about a diagnosis of HIV/ AIDS? What is the exact extent of a patient's right to know?

On the one hand, one could argue that a patient has exactly such a right-to-know on the general grounds of informed consent; that is, the patient is entitled to information not only about the risks of specific tests or treatments but about other dimensions of health care that might also pose risks.[6] Given the unavoidable cultural equation between HIV and death, we are not surprised that some persons who do not believe themselves to be otherwise at risk of HIV infection want to ensure that they avoid all possibility of infection at the hands of known or anonymous health-care providers. Other psychological motives might also prompt individuals to try to avoid health workers with HIV, including beliefs, for example, that such workers could be diminished in mental and physical skills or that they might also be compromised by drug use. Patients might also have moral and psychological preferences to avoid relationships with gay and bisexual men in whom HIV/AIDS is disproportionately prevalent. Seen as a matter of informed consent relevant to risk avoidance, HIV infection in a health worker should be disclosed as a matter of patient right. Some health-care workers encounter exactly such inquiries from patients.[7]

On the other hand, health workers have no obvious obligation to disclose all information a patient might seek. In order to feel comfortable with their physicians, patients might seek, for example, personal information about race, marriage, children, religion, or political beliefs. Such information is excludable from the standards of informed consent because it has no bearing on the capacity of the physician to carry out a particular procedure. By itself such information is extraneous to matters of diagnosis and treatment. Even if one limits inquiries to matters of risk attendant to medical treatment, it would be impossible to disclose all the relevant information that might affect the care of a particular individual, his or her treatment outcome, or the decision whether to accept care from a particular provider. Some commentators have, of course, noted that it is even laughable to expect full disclosure regarding all conceivable risks possible in the course of health care, else health practitioners would even have obligations to disclose risks of falls in the hospital or automobile accidents on the way to the hospital.[8] Certainly there are risks that ought to be disclosed, but ethics does not require endless, full disclosure regarding all risks possible in health care, even if some particular disclosure would in fact change a patient's decision. It is a matter of debate, of course, exactly what information ought to be disclosed as a matter of informed consent. But by itself an HIV/AIDS diagnosis is not a risk per se because the condition is not necessarily communicable; an HIV/AIDS diagnosis is thus just a piece of information about an individual. So the question about disclosure of HIV/AIDS diagnoses cannot be justified merely by a patient's wish to know or by an *expectation* of infection. The morally relevant question is whether HIV infection in a health-care provider belongs to the domain of risks that must ordinarily be disclosed or to the domain of risks whose remoteness does not oblige their disclosure, especially when expected treatment does not involve procedures—for example, those exposure-prone procedures as defined by the CDC[9]—in which accidents could end in exposure of a patient to a health-care worker's body fluids.

I am convinced that HIV infection in a health worker belongs to the domain of risks that do not ordinarily have to be disclosed to patients. First, accidental infection of patients is *rare in the extreme*. As mentioned in chapter 5, only five cases of infection of this kind have been reported and those were limited to the practice of a single dentist. There may have, of course, been other cases impossible to detect, for example, in persons whose infection in the course of health care was masked by the existence of another risk factor. A gay man, for example, may have become infected through a health-care provider's actions but he may also have practiced anal intercourse; confirming infection by a health worker could thus be confounded by the existence of multiple, possible means of infection. But the number of known cases of infection attributable to health workers is small—even minute—relative to the occurrence of HIV infection through other known means of infection: sex, needle-use, and blood transfusion. Given the extent of the HIV epidemic between 1980 and 1994, infection via an HIV-infected health worker represents the least significant means of HIV infection both in terms of total prevalence and incidence, and such a means of infection has not been identified as a risk linked either to specific patient populations, to specific treatment practices, or to specific classes of health workers. As a tiny and evidently late-occurring—and it appears at this point isolated—percentage of the total number of cases of HIV infection, especially when measured against the total number of health-care interventions in which such infection might have occurred during the period 1980–1994, accidental infection by a health worker represents a negligible risk to any given patient currently receiving health care.

Second, there is no evidence that health workers carry HIV infection at any disproportionately high rate compared to one's possible sexual partners or needle-sharing partners considered as a class. Certainly there are health workers with HIV infection,[10] but nothing in the reports of HIV infection or in prevalence studies suggests that *as a class* health workers pose a significantly higher rate of HIV infection than one might encounter in one's sexual partners or needle-sharing habits. For these reasons, we may conclude that health workers do not represent an "infected pool" whose communicable disease can be expected to cross inevitably or even commonly to patients in their care. Given increasing attention to safety precautions in medical care, HIV infection by a health worker has been and may be expected to remain—a rare occurrence in the United States. Setting aside as impossible a doctrine of full disclosure—whatever that might mean—a limited standard of disclosure would not therefore seem to require that health workers disclose any HIV/AIDS diagnosis as a matter of risk any more than they would be required to report other highly unusual, unexpected risks that could conceivably occur in the course of health care.

Even if the risk of infection by health-care workers is ordinarily negligible, one might argue that the serious consequences of infection alone justify disclosure. Even if the risk is statistically slight, AIDS is a syndrome of grave magnitude, and HIV infection by a health worker has already taken its first death.[11] The severity of AIDS may be granted, but it still does not follow logically that the only way to avoid HIV risk in health-care relations is through disclosure by workers of their own diagnoses. In response to patients' worries about HIV infection, health-care workers should indeed offer information about risks in the course of medical care, but that information need not include disclosure of their own HIV-related conditions. It is this distinction between risk disclosure and disclosure of individual diagnoses that I think should determine informed consent procedures in the area of HIV/AIDS, a point to which I will return after considering other aspects of the argument for the patient's generalized right-to-know.

Acknowledging a patient's right-to-know affects not only the patient's interests, for the interests of health workers are at stake as well. A patient's right-to-know might well jeopardize the interests of a health worker in a job and social setting. For example, health care in a contemporary hospital is typically provided by a range of persons from a variety of medical specialties. In surgical settings patients may not even be aware of all the persons on whom treatment depends, especially if a patient is unconscious during surgery. Patients are therefore often not able to identify all the persons involved in their health care. They might directly confront persons whom they can identify as their caregivers about personal HIV/AIDS diagnoses, but they will not be able to identify them all. Acknowledging a right to ascertain HIV infection then would have the effect of subjecting some health workers to constant inquiry about their health even as other health workers escaped this interrogation altogether. And it is worth wondering what form this kind of patient inquiry would take. Under what circumstances would a patient ask health workers about a possible HIV infection? At bedside examinations surrounded by medical students, interns, pharmacists, and hospital ethicists? In the hall surrounded by passersby, employers, and gossips? Recognizing the right of patients to ascertain HIV infection would not by itself mean that a patient had the right in any circumstances to inquire about and obtain that information. But without a policy of routine testing of all health workers and without formal assurance by health administrators (or private health workers) at one discrete, discreet point in a patient's health care about all the persons who will be involved in that care, exercising a putative right to such information can only be *random* and, moreover, potentially damaging in its consequences, not only to individual health workers but also to institutions whose reputations might suffer inappropriately from unintentional consequences of free-ranging inquiries about HIV/AIDS in their personnel.[12]

It is also worth looking at one other issue in the disclosure debate: the meaning of test results. A diagnosis of HIV represents a permanent condition since there is no cure for such an infection. Yet there is no symmetrical meaning for a health care worker found by testing to be uninfected. An HIV test has no predictive power; it reports—with a certain degree of accuracy—the infections it does or does not find in blood samples at a given time. Even if an individual tested him- or herself at regular intervals, still he or she might be unaware of an infection subsequently acquired. A patient's right-to-know could not therefore, even if acknowledged, guarantee patients freedom from care at the hands of people with HIV. This limitation of testing is not by itself any definitive argument that health-care workers ought not disclose their diagnoses, but it does show that any systematic attempt to undertake full disclosure would not be able to deliver what patients might expect. Such limitations do raise the interesting question of whether it is moral to assert a claim to disclosure when the nature of that disclosure cannot identify all health workers with HIV. Thus considered, the nonpredictive nature of HIV testing represents a buttressing consideration why a claimed right-to-know should be resisted, especially when protection from unwanted risk can be reasonably achieved in other ways.

What May a Patient Ask?

Physicians and other health workers may for reasons of their own choosing offer information to patients about a personal HIV/AIDS diagnosis. Some health workers *may want to and have in fact disclosed* such information if they believe that confirmation of their HIV/AIDS diagnosis would improve the quality of their relation with patients. A physician with a large clientele of people with AIDS, for example, might want to disclose an HIV diagnosis in order to reassure patients about his or her own understanding of their circumstances or commitment to their care. On the other hand, given the way in which certain physicians have lost their jobs[13] and their practices following such disclosures—whether such disclosures were voluntary or not—it is entirely understandable that only health workers who feel their interests adequately protected in regard to employment, insurability, and social circumstance would be inclined to confirm freely an HIV/AIDS diagnosis to patients.

Perhaps rejecting a patient's right-to-know on the grounds that it is prejudicial to workers leaves behind the sense that only their confidentiality matters. Perhaps there is the sentiment that rejecting a right to demand disclosure is insensitive to the needs of patient protection. It does not follow, though, from these arguments that patients must enter blind into risks in their treatment. On the contrary, there are adequate moral foundations for standards of patient protection already recognized even if specific practices in regard to HIV risks are not widely followed. The same moral (and legal) incentives that guide risk disclosure in regard to medical therapies and experiments extend—though not without limit—to risk disclosure about possible HIV infection in the course of health care. These standards of informed consent offer patients acceptable protection against risks of HIV infection. In addition, adequate information can be provided to a patient without disclosure of the HIV/AIDS status of any single health worker. For example, a person anticipating hernia surgery may appropriately ask his health-care providers what treatments he will undergo that might expose him to accidental HIV transmission from any of the health workers involved in his care. A physician's response to such an inquiry would presumably involve details about the known occurrence of HIV infection in health-care settings, the extent to which the proposed surgery is susceptible to accidental infection, the number of health workers involved in his care and their experience, the precautions that will be taken to prevent accidental exposure, and even possible options for treatment or experimental therapy should there be an accidental "bleed" of a health worker during surgery. This kind of detail is already long familiar in informed consent protocols in medicine. Thus informed, the patient can decide whether to accept the surgery *without* having to identify an HIV/AIDS diagnosis in each and every individual involved in his care and *without* having to ascertain that information in a haphazard and potentially prejudicial way. Some individuals might find the risks unacceptable; if a physician stumbles in explaining the degree of risk, standards of protection, or options following accidental exposure, a patient may decide that he is unwilling to submit to HIV risk in this health-care setting and take his hernia needs elsewhere. Because of personal experience and institutional support some physicians have already instituted high standards of care to avoid accidental exposure. They may additionally be involved in experimental protocols of drug therapy designed specifically to prevent HIV infection from taking hold in patients accidentally exposed. This kind of planned effort would undoubtedly prove attractive to persons concerned about accidental HIV infection.

Health care obviously cannot always be provided under conditions that permit exquisitely detailed conversations about risks and precautions, and much medical care is provided to patients whose conditions do not permit medical window shopping. For example, a patient entering an emergency room unconscious, bleeding, and without friends or relatives at hand is not in a position to conduct informed consent interviews let alone worry about protection from iatrogenic HIV infection. And persons who receive health care at public institutions for the reason alone that they have no other means of health care are typically not able to walk away from risks they perceive in those institutions. Moreover, psychological or cultural reasons having to do with intimidation by doctors or language barriers might impede aggressive inquiry about HIV risks. In view of these kinds of circumstances, a general policy of informed consent alone would still not permit people to avoid unwanted associations with HIV/AIDS risk. Such limitations on informed consent, however, do not amount to convincing reasons for asserting an unconditional right-to-know. The inability of specific individuals to take advantage of the benefits of informed consent does not diminish informed consent as an ideal. And in any case these same limitations in the practice of informed consent would also function as limitations on any legislated right to ascertain information about HIV/AIDS in one's health-care providers.

Another issue involved in the disclosure/consent debate is the role of concealment in jeopardizing the health-care relationship. Suspicion of one's health-care providers might prove a powerful corrosive in these delicate relations, and certainly the argument for disclosure raises the specter of patients and health workers circling one another with mutual suspicion, thereby undermining the desired atmosphere of trust and the assumption of mutual benefit. Such a development could easily take place anyway, given the unequal relations that obtain between the sick and the well, between the medically uninformed and the medically educated, especially when these divisions are deepened by stratifications of class, race, gender, and sexual orientation. Yet because of the design and delivery of health care in the United States today and because of a moral presumption of patient and physician autonomy, a certain adversarial component to health-care relations may be inevitable and even beneficial. Physician and philosopher H. Tristam Engelhardt, Jr., has described many of the reasons why patients find themselves "strangers in a strange land," and he explains the burden health-care providers face in regard to disclosure of an expected course of medical experience.[14] Unfortunate as it may sound, some consumer awareness must come from the person seeking health care. Health care is typically provided by a wide variety of persons and institutions in a wide spectrum of specialties, responsibilities, economic loyalties, and even geographies. If only by default, in order to sort out the landscape of health-care systems, patients must assume certain responsibilities in seeking health care consonant with their needs, interests, and economics. We cannot assume automatically that all health workers or institutions have only the best interests of every individual patient at the center of decision-making. Patients, therefore, must be understood as having a certain responsibility toward their own lives and health interests. Such a presumption of autonomy also highlights the risk of patient infantilizing which could occur were health workers alone to bear the responsibility for a patient's health. While informed consent may be difficult to achieve, its focus on the risks of treatments and on remedies for such risks remains a worthy regulatory ideal to be observed in health relations.

One related reason for rejecting a patient's right-to-know comes from the nature of the obligation a person has to protect himself or herself. I assume that people ordinarily have a general obligation to protect themselves from harm, certainly from the kind of harm HIV infection brings. Such an obligation may be intensified if the individual is committed to the care and protection of others in, say, assuming responsibilities for family members. This general obligation, however, may also be suspended for adequate reason; we do not consider it immoral that people commit themselves to military service in time of just war, for example, or otherwise jeopardize their lives for altruistic motives. This general obligation to protect oneself is therefore not the only obligation a person has. Nor does this general obligation require that a person protect against *all* possible risk. Life in contemporary society virtually requires accepting some risks that jeopardize life and health, for example, driving in Boston or crossing a Chicago street. Given the known, low occurrence of accidental HIV infection it is not obvious that anyone could claim a right to be protected from that risk by means of compelling disclosure of HIV infection in any and all health care personnel. No one has the *obligation* to protect himself or herself to that degree.

Philosopher John Rawls, in his *A Theory of Justice*, presents a heuristic device for imagining how fairness of access and opportunity in social policy and social goods might be achieved.[15] This device of the "original position," in which principles of social governance are formulated without specific knowledge of the role one would actually have in society, may be used as one last way to think about the social entitlements of health-care workers with HIV infections. If persons charged with formulating policy regarding patient access to HIV/AIDS diagnosis in health workers did not themselves know their HIV status, it would be in their interests to create policy that protected both patients and health workers from HIV risk *as well as* from capricious disclosure of medical diagnoses. A policy of informed consent as to risks and barriers to risk seems likely to emerge as the consensus from such a policy-making group. Patients would gain thereby the right to identify all the risks of their particular treatment and decide for themselves whether there would be adequate protection from those risks, and health workers would gain thereby protection from involuntary disclosure of medical diagnoses and be able to remain to exercise their skills in their chosen occupations.

One last consideration worth mentioning in regard to an HIV right-to-know is that this right may assume a prejudicial entitlement when not equivalently sought or recognized in regard to other health-worker characteristics, such as alcohol and drug use, surgery success rates, history of epilepsy, civil and criminal prosecutions, and so on down the list of human frailties and venalities that might affect the outcome of a particular medical intervention. To the extent other features of health-care workers are not sought out as a matter of informed consent, does not inquiry in regard to HIV assume that HIV infection is a greater risk than any other kind of risk involved in medical care? Does not the right-to-know argument carry with it the implication that except for health-care risks patients would not otherwise be at risk of HIV? The conceptual framework behind an insistence on a right-to-know implies that HIV is confined to a certain class of individuals and that the so-called general population is otherwise free of risk. This expectation is not only untrue to the facts of HIV infection but carries with it the morally questionable conceptual tools by which to distinguish "innocent" HIV/AIDS from culpable HIV/AIDS.

The Accidental Exposure

Suppose, for reasons unforeseen by anyone, a surgeon with an HIV infection—he is without clinical symptoms though he does take anti-HIV drugs—by accident cuts through his gloves and bleeds into a patient's abdominal cavity during surgery. Suppose, moreover, that the bleeding is quickly controlled and the blood suctioned off as thoroughly as possible. What obligation does the surgeon have to disclose this information to the patient? As mentioned earlier, there is always the voluntary option of a health worker to disclose infection to a patient, and some physicians in this circumstance might wish to disclose the event to the patient. But does the physician have any moral *obligation* to disclose under such circumstances?

An obligation to disclose a "mistake" that may end in a patient's infection depends on several arguments, most of which arise from a general presumption of beneficence toward the patient and monitoring a patient's health. First of all, the physician's obligation to guide a patient through the postoperative period and monitor any pathological developments is understood as morally unproblematic. To the extent that an HIV-related condition might be a postoperative development in a patient following a bleeding accident, a surgeon then has the duty to warn the patient that such conditions may occur and the patient ought to be instructed about what to look for in this regard. Second, some patients might wish to enroll in an experimental program of drug treatment in the hope of preventing an inoculum of HIV from effecting a true infection. Such programs have now been carried out after occupational needle-stick injuries, for example, although their efficacy is far from certain.[16] Insofar as a patient's participation in such a program depends on timely notification of exposure, disclosure becomes paramount. This rationale would be diminished to the extent to which no experimental drug protocol is available or intended. Time and research may prove such experimental interventions are beneficial; to the extent they are *not*, this latter arm of the argument for disclosure would dissolve.

To argue from the heuristic of Rawls's original position, perhaps such a duty is owed the patient, not on consequentialist grounds necessarily, but as a matter of respect to the patient and as disclosure that all similarly situated persons would reasonably expect and want to know. This understanding might well be the consensus of a group in the original position. But there is nothing in the nature of these disclosures that requires the person with HIV to be named. To be sure, sometimes the circumstances of the medical treatment will make it obvious who the infected party is, but in a multiperson surgical team the infected team member is not always obvious. Knowing the specific identity of the member of the health-care team with HIV/AIDS would be of no benefit in terms of monitoring oneself for the development of an HIV-related condition or enrollment in experimental drugs trials. Only a claim that HIV infection resulted from *wrongful* behavior on the part of a health worker would justify disclosure of the identity of the health worker with HIV/AIDS insofar as an injured patient wished to charge negligence as the cause of the accidental exposure.

Accidental HIV infection does, of course, raise important questions regarding the uses of the law. In matters of tort, the law is certainly interested in at least two areas relevant to accidental HIV infection: HIV risks that belong to negligent medical care and HIV risks that follow failure to inform. These concerns may be pursued in litigation either jointly or separately. In the first instance the law upholds sanctions with respect to medical care that was not competently provided and that resulted in personal injury. In the second instance the law also countenances sanctions against health workers not specifically because injury occurs—some iatrogenic injury, after all, is unpreventable even when treatment is entirely competent—but because information about that possible injury was not disclosed and thus an individual's right to avoid treatment was usurped.[17] The law may thus concern itself with patient HIV infection in at least these ways: first, it may impose sanctions against negligent medical care that ended in HIV infection of a patient. Because such legal action asserts negligent behavior, not failure to disclose per se, it might succeed even though a health worker did not disclose his or her own HIV-related condition prior to the negligent treatment. The success of cases of negligence therefore do not appear to depend on prior disclosure and for purposes of this essay the case for the right-to-know is not bolstered by an appeal to the workings of tort law.

Second, a case that proceeds on the grounds that patient choice was controlled—to his or her detriment—by a health worker's failure to disclose a personal HIV-related condition might succeed at trial. If the patient in the surgery scenario discussed above did develop an HIV infection and then claimed that he or she could have—or would have—chosen another surgeon given notice of the surgeon's HIV infection, then the court might wish to sanction such a health worker or hospital in some way. In fact, some courts have held that physicians and their employing institutions ought to have disclosed HIV infections to patients prior to any medical treatment. The nature of damages appropriate to such "lapses" has been contested, but some courts have recognized damages even where the patients involved did not themselves incur an HIV infection.[18] Yet for all the reasons I have offered here, such a conclusion should be generally resisted; that is, the remote possibility of exposure and infection should not open the door to an unlimited obligation to disclose HIV/AIDS diagnoses. Additionally, a legally recognized subjective standard requiring health workers to disclose all information that could cause a patient to seek treatment elsewhere would "constitute a severe burden for physicians who would need to show that they had satisfied the worries of particular patients. There would always be the temptation for a patient to consider after the fact that the physician had not dealt with one of the patient's special concerns,"[19] as Tristam Engelhardt has observed.

The possibility of resort to law may in itself produce significant incentives for physicians and hospitals to define and adhere to effective prophylactic techniques.[20] This would certainly be desirable, but of course we cannot know to what extent the expectation of lawsuits will limit accidental HIV exposure in health care. Nor is it certain that disclosure of HIV/AIDS status by a health worker prior to treatment would shield that worker from all tort liability in the event of a subsequent negligent or accidental infection. Given then the difficulty in establishing that in fact a patient would have sought out another surgeon, given that informed consent procedures afford the opportunity of identifying and accepting HIV risks, given that iatrogenic HIV infection is a remote risk, given that tort remedies may apply, the patient ought not to expect disclosure about HIV infection in health workers as a matter of course.

This conclusion does not suggest lack of concern about accidental HIV infection of a patient. Rather, it says that *both* informed consent relative to the risks of HIV infection *and* professional and institutional efforts to identify effective HIV barriers throughout the entire domain of health care will do more to prevent accidental HIV infection than occasional legal sanctions—with unknown deterrent effect—against a few health workers whose negligence or accidents end in HIV infections in their patients. Nevertheless, because of uncertainty about how courts will respond to claims about the failure of health workers to inform patients of personal HIV/AIDS diagnoses, affected health workers may find it prudent to voluntarily withdraw from exposure-prone procedures whose safety cannot be assured.[21] It may even be that health workers who perform exposure-prone treatments have a moral obligation to monitor themselves voluntarily for HIV infection[22] and impairment of professional skill. But it is worth noting here again that this kind of monitoring and withdrawal can take place without disclosure of personal HIV/AIDS diagnoses.

My arguments thus far apply as well to so-called "look back" notification, that is, retrospective notification of patients that one of their health workers has been identified with HIV/AIDS. The state of Illinois, for example, authorized in 1991 (1) notification of those patients who had undergone invasive treatment procedures by a health worker subsequently diagnosed with HIV/AIDS and (2) notification of health workers when patients were similarly identified. I do not agree that patients have a general right to such notification unless some specific negligent behavior is known to have occurred or unless some nonnegligent means of accidental infection has been identified that either led to infection or was likely to do so. In any case, disclosure of this kind need not disclose which health worker has HIV/AIDS, though in some cases it will be impossible to protect personal identity.

The question of rights in regard to information about individual health workers is, of course, one that recapitulates many of the central questions about the HIV epidemic at this time. Certainly, the epidemic has blurred distinctions between private and public.[23] But dissolving the private into the public will not by itself halt the epidemic. On the contrary, the protection of the private can permit health workers with HIV/AIDS to retain control of their life interests amid a swirl of interpretations and judgments made about their lives as a "threat" to public health. The need to protect the realm of the private can also spur inventiveness in health-care settings if what is necessary to protect patients is not disclosure but prophylaxis. One way to read the appeal of a right-to-know for patients is to understand it as expressing fear of health-care institutions and workers. Thus construed, assuring safe health care, regardless of the type of institution or the medical conditions of individual health workers, ought to be the primary moral concern in adopting standards and policies that make people unafraid to seek health care. Such a concern would emerge as the chief consideration too from any Rawlsian original position group assembled to identify the relative priorities of means of controlling HIV infection in health-care settings. Certainly, professional agencies and health institution administrations should protect patients from substandard or negligent care related to HIV-related disability. Some patients, in fact, might not necessarily fear infection from their health-care providers but might fear impaired treatment from infected health-care workers as the result of the mental and physical disabilities associated with HIV pathogenesis and HIV drug treatment. Such a concern is, of course, fair to address in all health workers, not only those with HIV-related conditions. And because such a concern is universal, special precautions should be taken to insure patients that care will not be substandard by reason of any health worker impairment. Nonetheless, fairness demands that no special tests should be required for such workers which are not equally imposed on health workers for possible impairment by reason of alcohol use, drug use, senescence, emotional disability, and similar problems. There is nothing about the nature of impairments associated with HIV that requires special tests whose goal is more to "purify" health care than to protect actual patients from real situations of risk. Whatever standards an institution might have for identifying impairment in health-care workers could also be disclosed, when requested, in informed consent processes. The possibility of this disclosure—and the protection it makes possible in patient choice—serves therefore as a final reason why no patient right-to-know about individual health worker's diagnoses with HIV/AIDS should be recognized even as it highlights the importance of both individual and institutional vigilance necessary for patient protection.

7

Teaching AIDS in China

The significance of cultural mores for AIDS prevention in the medical setting was underlined for me by a visit to the People's Republic of China. In January 1992 for a month, I taught in a master's program the University of Illinois was offering at Beijing Medical University. With Illinois faculty traveling to Beijing for a number of three- and four-week sessions, the university offered its Master's of Health Professions Education degree during a period from 1991 to 1992. This degree is designed for health professionals who find themselves unprepared for educational and leadership responsibilities they assume or seek in the course of their professional careers. This program offers instruction in research design, testing and evaluation methods, curriculum development, topics in contemporary medical education, educational leadership, and medical humanities, with various options in electives and thesis requirements. It is the only such degree program in the United States.

In that master's program I have offered instruction and discussion in ethics, focusing on ethical concerns faced by individual health professionals and by society at large in its health-care policies. Because the students in the China program were mostly physicians who held educational and administrative responsibilities, I found it especially interesting to look at the question of HIV/AIDS against the backdrop of the political, ethical, and health-care standards of that country. This opportunity also offered me another perspective on formulating health-care policy, for I had just served at the University of Illinois Hospital as a member of a committee charged with determining policy for university health-care workers with HIV.

Professor Zero

Because I had never been to China and did not know how discussion of AIDS, sexuality, drug use, and similar topics would be received there, I had a certain uneasiness about exporting components of my own "AIDS and Ethics" course to China. I was also not sure that the students would already have or develop an interest in the epidemic that has so entangled the United States and many other regions of the world. In this regard I felt like "Professor Zero,"[1] the teacher who was bringing AIDS to Chinese classrooms whether it was wanted there or not. I expected the experience to be unlike my teaching at the University of Illinois, where I can presume that students *expect* discussions of HIV/AIDS in ethical issues facing health care. I also planned to address ethical dilemmas familiar to the Chinese in their own health-care system: resource allocation, euthanasia, maldistribution of physicians, and other problems similar to those encountered in the United States. I used a number of essays written by Chinese scholars on exactly those topics. I wanted, however, with my instruction about HIV/AIDS to offer certain American perspectives and to set these Chinese physicians thinking about what their own society's response could and should be.

My first encounter with Chinese attitudes toward AIDS occurred on the plane. En route from Narita airport near Tokyo to China, passengers were given forms to fill out, including the "Passenger's Health Declaration." On that form passengers were asked to indicate any current illness, including the following conditions: "Psychosis, Leprosy, AIDS (inc. AIDS virus carrier), Venereal Diseases, Active Pulmonary Diseases." Passengers were also queried about bleeding, vomiting, diarrhea, jaundice, or lymph-gland swelling. The same form inquired whether passengers were carrying old clothes, which, I presumed, were suspected of possible infestation.

Whether an inquiry like this—one form among others handed to weary travelers distracted by their own concerns—could achieve the goal of preventing the unauthorized entry into China of anyone with HIV/AIDS is questionable. Anyone with the savvy required to book a flight to China from the United States, obtain a visa, and negotiate the sprawl of international airports would ordinarily have the sophistication required to lie about his or her condition. Unless the reason for the Chinese question about AIDS is to gather evidence of fraud to use in subsequent deportation of persons later discovered to have HIV/ AIDS, the questionnaire—negligently and mechanically collected at Beijing customs by a bored young man in drab military dress—seems to be but a gesture, something to be held out that the government is in fact doing something to protect its nation from threats it holds to be exogenous. In this regard, we may wonder to what extent nationalism impedes an appreciation of the global character of the HIV epidemic.

China's social and political history give a special resonance to the question of excluding foreign nationals with HIV. The formidable Great Wall of China, dating from the third century B.C.E., and the historical preoccupation of China with controlling the movements of people within and across its borders is a dramatic background against which to consider that country's efforts in regard to HIV control, especially as HIV is viewed as a problem of foreigners. While once visiting the Great Wall, Jonathan Mann, now director of the International AIDS Center at Harvard, asked his Chinese hosts, "Did it work—that Wall?" The answer he got from members of the Chinese Ministry of Health acknowledged that AIDS cannot be stopped by exclusionary walls. As Mann notes, "Walls represent a danger of isolation, not a source of protection."[2] Lessons elsewhere around the globe show that HIV/ AIDS is too important a problem to relegate to the margins for very long, whether those margins are social or geographical.

AIDS in China

China first reported a case of AIDS in 1985, at a time when the United States already had more than twelve thousand reported cases.[3] One measure of the current interpretation of AIDS in China at the time of my visit may be taken from its official English-language newspaper, *China Daily*. This government-controlled paper is filled with headlines and articles about improvements of all kinds across China. Its reports tout control of crime, improvement of factory production, expansion of international academic ties, and the newest movies about the successful "re-education" of Chiang Kai-shek soldiers who failed to escape the mainland. The paper also typically features a story or two about disasters and/or political turbulence around the world; stories on American crime and scandal loom large here. Its message is otherwise doggedly upbeat.

On December 2, 1991, that newspaper ran a story, "China Seen Alert and Active on World Aids Day," which reported that "China is keeping a close eye on the spread of AIDS in the country and is taking stringent measures to control it, according to a senior health official." Reporting on activities surrounding World AIDS day, the article revealed that since 1985

China has found 8 sufferers and 607 infected by the Aids virus in 15 provinces, cities, and autonomous regions. Among them are three mainland Aids sufferers, one of whom had just returned from abroad. He was found to have been infected by the AIDS virus in 1989 and died in July this year. The Aids-infected are mainly drug addicts in the southwestern border regions, people in inland provinces who have returned from abroad where they have been working as part of an exported workforce, people in coastal areas who have returned from visits abroad, and prostitutes in the big cities.[4]

The use of "sufferers" here indicates that at least someone associated with the paper is aware of the controversy about labels applied to people with AIDS and has forsworn in this instance the prejudicial and self-fulfilling aspects of the term "AIDS victim," even if using a euphemism does its own damage.[5] Yet, the same article did use the term "AIDS victim" elsewhere and in doing so joined the ranks of papers worldwide which continue to use this term not to underline the accidental nature of HIV infection but to emphasize the medical and social plight of PWAs[6] if not also to position them as responsible for that plight.

Whatever the occurrence of HIV/AIDS may be in China[7] and whatever the Chinese choose to call people with AIDS, the representation in this press account parallels accounts of the beginning of AIDS in other places.[8] HIV/AIDS has generally been characterized as a condition whose origins are located in drug use and sexual immorality and, in the case of Chinese accounts, in regions outside China itself. HIV/AIDS is therefore representable as a condition whose origins belong, at best, to personal weakness or, at worst, to antisocial immorality. It is interesting that this report makes no explicit mention of homosexuality, a highly significant omission, given the association of AIDS with homosexuality in the Americas and Europe, a point to which I will return later.

AIDS in the Classroom

The twenty-nine Chinese students in the Illinois program were almost all physicians, ranging in age from twenty-four to forty-one. They typically had some form of administrative responsibility in their institutions throughout China for health professions education, whether in medicine, nursing, or pharmacy. The few students who were not physicians were all employed by medical universities in one capacity or another; one student, for example, was a pharmacist charged with redesigning his school's graduate curriculum in pharmacy. Only a few students had been abroad; only one had ever been to the United States. Their skill in understanding and speaking English was typically quite good; some had attended the English-speaking medical universities in China. Facility in English had, in any case, been a condition of admission to the program. None of the instructors spoke more than a few words of Chinese.

Partly as an introduction to ethics in the United States and partly as an example of how courses in medical humanities are conducted at the University of Illinois, I showed my students a slide collection that I use for discussion in my own "AIDS and Ethics" class. All the students had heard of AIDS and shared the view that the problem of AIDS in China was small and confined mainly to provinces in the south of the country associated with drug trade. After offering a few introductory remarks about the nature of AIDS, its prevalence in the United States according to CDC figures, and the principal mechanisms of HIV infection, I presented slides of medical, educational, and activist images of the epidemic.

The slides were taken from various sources. I used a few slides from biomedical journals: electron microscopy photographs, molecular drawings, a green monkey, and even a beautifully colored crystal of Retrovir, a drug used to treat people with AIDS. I also presented a number of slides of posters from around the world which presented AIDS in fearful if not also moralistic ways. I used, for example, the cover of an issue of the *Medical Journal of Australia* which carried an x-ray of lungs affected by *Pneumocystis carinii* pneumonia, a skull and shroud, and the enquiry: "Perhaps we've needed a situation like this to confirm what we've known all along—depravity kills."[9] I also used reproductions from *AIDS: Images for Survival*, a collection of AIDS poster art that abounds in skulls and flaming heads and bloody pistols and other images of fear and death, among them, for example, a flaming red head bearing the caption "Mr. Aids would love to meet you"[10] (see figure 2).

Against the backdrop of such fear-evoking images I also presented a number of slides of AIDS activist origin. I used reproductions of images in Douglas Crimp's anthology *AIDS: Cultural Analysis/Cultural Activism* and Crimp and Adam Rolston's *AIDS Demo Graphics*.[11] Using images of their own making, AIDS activists have challenged the automatic equation of AIDS and death and have substituted other equations altogether, as in the case of the widely known black poster SILENCE = DEATH, which recalls with its pink triangle the Nazi internment and extermination of gay men.[12] I also showed slides of activists being arrested and posters protesting social inaction and discrimination. "THE GOVERNMENT HAS BLOOD ON ITS HANDS" reads the legend for one widely circulated image of a bloody handprint (see figure 3). Some of the poster art I showed affirmed gay and lesbian sexuality against social interpretations that have equated such sexuality identity with death.[13] I also presented a number of slides of black-and-white photographs of people with HIV/AIDS from the collection *Epitaphs for the Living*[14] as well as photographs of textile memorials from *The Quilt: Stories from the Names Project*.

I took to China one poster—not just a slide—that has had a stormy history here in the United States. The poster depicts three couples kissing or on the verge of kissing. The three couples consist of a man and woman, two men, and two women (see figure 4). This poster was produced by Gran Fury, a New York activist art collective that grew out of the activist group ACT UP. The original legend for this poster read only: "Kissing doesn't kill. Greed and indifference do." But because the poster was misinterpreted in the United States to suggest that people's unwillingness to constrain their sexual desires led to AIDS, another line of text was added at the bottom of the poster to include a more specific indictment of the inaction attributed to government and the machinations of capitalist society: "Corporate Greed, Government, Inaction, and Public Indifference Make AIDS a Political Crisis."[15] When this poster was put up at various points in Chicago in 1990, it was sometimes ripped down or blackened over with paint by persons who opposed it. The mayor of the city called for "less offensive" ads,[16] and some Chicago aldermen even called a special meeting of the city

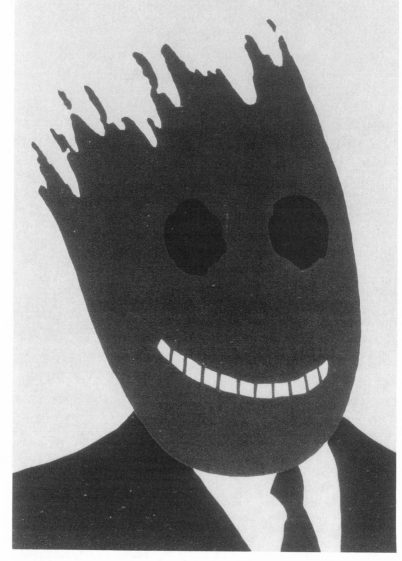

Mr. Aids
would love to meet you.

2. This fiery-headed anthropomorphization of AIDS suggests the immolating dangers of AIDS and evokes images of PWAs as hellish figures, even burning in hell. The smile, formal dress, and formal nomenclature bespeak the decorous images behind which AIDS may lurk. Though it incites a fearful response to AIDS, the poster does not offer any advice on how to protect oneself from AIDS. Poster originally appeared in Charles Helmken's *AIDS: Images for Survival* (Washington, D.C.: Shosin Society, 1989). Courtesy of the artist, Seymour Chwast.

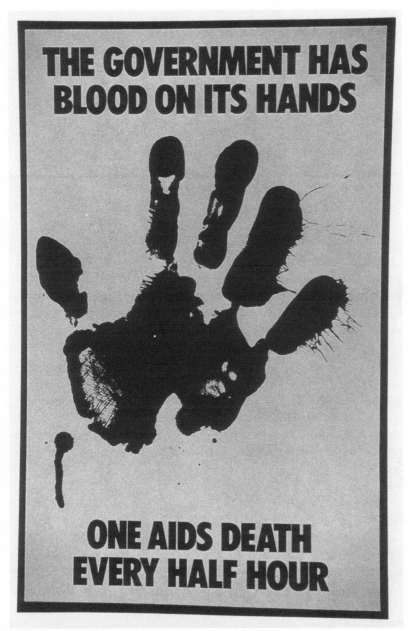

3. This simple, self-consciously provocative graphic rejects the view that PWAs have brought death on themselves. On the contrary, it declares that government—by unspecified means—is responsible for the mounting AIDS death toll. Courtesy of ACT UP.

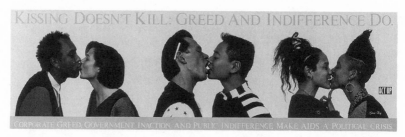

4. This poster of couples mixed by race and gender drew fire in Chicago for "promoting" homosexuality. Courtesy of Gran Fury.

council in an unsuccessful effort to "tear down these morally offensive posters."[17] The "promotion" of homosexuality was the chief complaint lodged against the posters and the endangerment of children was cited as its chief mischief.

A poster by "Gang," a New York art collective, varied the familiar Marlboro cigarette advertisements. One familiar American icon known throughout the world is the American cowboy, and the students laughed to see President George Bush represented as a cowboy, over a cigarette package-style warning that his administration could be hazardous to one's health because of its inaction on AIDS (see figure 5). The students laughed even more when I asked if they would be able to get away with producing a similar poster featuring their own prime minister, Li Peng. The students easily understood the message of these posters: that business and government were failing to do their parts against the epidemic. Perhaps this recognition should not be surprising in a country where health care is provided as a matter of political doctrine by government. Unfortunately, the message about safety in the "Kissing Doesn't Kill" poster was, as in the U.S., misconstrued.

I lingered on each of these slides as long as class attention seemed to warrant, but there was not as much discussion by the students as I would have liked. Part of the reason for this lack of participation stems from the Chinese educational system, which does not promote classroom discussion between students and teachers, even in higher education. My colleagues and I found this reluctance to participate in discussion a frequent frustration, yet as far as I could tell from the students who did speak, the slides were well received. The students were interested in the images—and the social climate that allowed such sharp criticism of government—and they were quick to understand some of

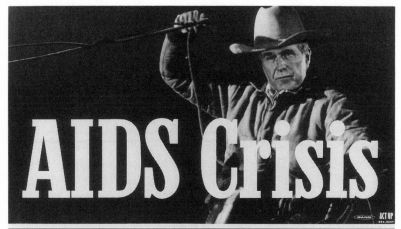

AVISO: Mientras que Bush gasta billones jugando a vaquero, 37 millones de norte americanos no tienen seguro medico. Un norte americano muere de SIDA cada ocho minutos.

5. This satire of a widely recognized cigarette advertisement depicts President George Bush in the macho pose of the cowboy of American folklore. The caption reads: "Warning: While Bush wastes billions playing cowboy, 37 million North Americans have no medical insurance. A North American dies of AIDS every eight minutes." The billions of dollars refers to the money used to finance the military in general and the Persian Gulf war in particular. Reprinted by permission of Gang.

the issues that have engaged AIDS education here in the United States. They noted, for example, that many AIDS posters did equate HIV with death and that while some posters warn against the grave nature of AIDS they do not equivalently educate people about what measures they should take to protect themselves. For example, one poster showed a male hand poised to masturbate accompanied by the legend: "This Might Be Your Best Friend."[18] Some people might be scared into a life of masturbation by AIDS, but most will not and for those persons the poster has no educational message at all about safety in sex. Though I had less feedback than I would have liked about the slides, the students appeared to understand not only the overt messages of the images but also their political implications. Interpreting implicit messages of poster art is not an unfamiliar task for the Chinese. Abundant political posters and slogans are a way of life in their country. Around the city of Beijing, for example, numerous political messages appear on large billboards with the message in both Chinese and English: "Practice Family Planning. Implement the National Priority."

AIDS Assignment

Apart from discussion of these visual representations of AIDS, I assigned students to determine a policy for the Murphy General Hospital for health-care workers diagnosed with HIV/AIDS. "Specifically," the assignment read, "you are asked to determine (*a*) whether health-care workers should be tested for HIV as a matter of employment or review and (*b*) whether any restrictions on patient care should be adopted for health-care workers with HIV infections or disease, and if so, how such restrictions should be adopted and enforced." The problem offered a number of points of convergence in a curriculum devoted to ethical as well as to theoretical and practical aspects of leadership and management. To prepare their recommendations the students divided into four groups. Other faculty members and I circulated among the groups as resource personnel, often role-playing parts as hospital administrators, deans of medical schools, ministers of public health, and so on.

After a number of meetings, the groups reported back to the whole class. The reports shared a number of conclusions. Every group pointed out the importance of protecting the hospital's reputation in order to make it attractive to people and to assure patients of their safety. Too, the groups all suggested that some form of HIV testing take place, whether at initial employment or some point annually thereafter. One group thought that only persons involved in invasive procedures should be tested; testing others would be irrelevant. Only one person in all the groups thought that persons with HIV should be fired because of an HIV/AIDS diagnosis; despite the singularity of this view it was nonetheless expressed adamantly. All the groups also thought that a health worker discovered through testing to have an HIV infection should be transferred away from patient care or simply not hired. Two groups mentioned as a rationale for this policy the protection of *the workers* with HIV, that is, protecting *them* from illnesses borne by patients. Nevertheless, arguments focusing on protection of patients and reputation seemed to be the prevailing rationale for keeping health-care workers with HIV/AIDS separate from patients. Recalling the message of the slide they had seen earlier in the week which blamed inaction and failure to plan proactively for the epidemic, two groups ended their presentation by recalling that "Silence = Death" and urged the administrators of Murphy General Hospital to take swift action in implementing their recommendations.

These discussions and recommendations might have come from equivalent groups in the United States. The CDC, for example, has wrangled with the question of testing health workers whose work involves "invasive" or "exposure-prone" treatment measures.[19] And this is no idle question, especially in light of the HIV infections caused by the dentist David Acer. Questions of transfers—if not loss of employment—have also been discussed as matters relevant to patient protection from health workers with HIV/AIDS. So there was nothing extraordinary about the recommendations these Chinese health professionals made. The reasons for their recommendations may have varied slightly from those that might be offered in the United States, of course, but the students did not elaborate much—and neither was there much time for such elaboration—on their group rationales. One might imagine, though, that certain background issues, such as the social policy of full employment in the country, might have influenced their preferences for transferring rather than firing workers with HIV/AIDS.

But not only in recommendations did the Chinese discussion parallel the debate in the United States; the ensuing criticism of the Chinese proposals also sounded familiar themes. Not all the groups shared the same recommendations, and not every member in a group shared its majority consensus. Some individuals rejected policies of testing and transferring altogether. One physician in the class, for example, insistently pointed out that he would not want to accept a transfer merely for the sake of protecting a hospital's reputation if he had an HIV infection but was still able to perform his job. He would *especially* not want a transfer if his job did not entail risks to patients. As discussions with health workers with HIV/AIDS in the United States have shown, this reluctance is no personal quirk or selfish disregard of patient safety; on the contrary, the issue raises profound questions about standards of employment and limitations on interventions against people with HIV.

One other student also persistently challenged the merit of HIV testing of health workers, either at the time of initial employment or on an annual basis thereafter. Not a physician herself, she pointed out that such testing could not ensure that an individual would not develop an HIV infection *after* employment and that continuous testing—at intervals of once or even twice a year—would not ensure (*a*) accurate identification of health workers with HIV *or* for that reason (*b*) patient safety. She pointed out that testing would also increase costs to a health-care system burdened with other costs it could not now meet.

In the fall of 1991 I had served on the University of Illinois Hospital and Clinics Ad Hoc Committee for the formulation of policy regarding health workers with either HIV or hepatitis B virus (HBV) infection. (Like many other institutions at the time, the university formed this committee in reaction to widespread publicity about HIV infection by a health-care worker and in reaction to CDC recommendations about formulating guidelines on practice limitations for the HIV-infected health-care workers; the university was not reacting to any specific incident in its hospital or clinics or to the presence of HIV infection in a specific employee.) As I listened to the Chinese students, I was struck time and again by their raising of many of the issues that surfaced as concerns during the Illinois committee meetings; many of the same recommendations were advanced and many of the same criticisms of those proposals emerged. The university committee finally adopted a majority recommendation against instituting any kind of routine HIV/ HBV screening for its health workers (or even for employees not directly involved in patient care; this latter was a response to university attorney's concern for receptionist-patient interactions). The committee did recommend a policy that would make voluntary screening available to health workers. Furthermore, the committee adopted a policy that health workers who know themselves to have an HIV/HBV infection must report their diagnosis to their department head. The head of the department would then in turn convene a special University Hospital and Clinics advisory committee to review the worker's responsibilities and recommend any work limitations on a case-by-case basis, with every effort being made to protect the confidentiality and employability of the worker. Such a policy, of course, is open to criticism because it creates policy for HIV and HBV when it does not do so for other conditions that might jeopardize a patient's care, conditions like alcoholism, epilepsy, or depression. Such selective policy is morally problematic, certainly, because it not only singles out one condition but also because it leaves great latitude to the advisory committee regarding decisions about a worker's job responsibilities.[20] In their recommendations the Chinese students did not directly propose standards that obligated health workers to report HIV-related conditions to a supervisor, and neither did they raise the possibility of oversight committees that would make recommendations about the employment responsibilities of a health worker. But certainly incisive remarks they made about the limitations of testing and the problem of transferring health workers echo the issues raised by the Illinois hospital committee. Given more time for the assignment and more firsthand experience in dealing with the problem of HIV in health workers and patients, I do not doubt that the Chinese group of health professionals would eventually have raised issues of reporting and work assignments even if they came to different conclusions than did the committee in Chicago. That they did not raise such issues may be a result of the common perception that health workers with HIV is a remote concern in China at present. Many of the health professionals who come from the more remote provinces of China may in fact never see a person with AIDS let alone have to grapple with questions of the employability of an infected health-worker.

AIDS and Morality

Because my stay in China was limited and because my sampling of the views of the Chinese was anecdotal, I cannot claim to be presenting universal perceptions of the importance of the problem of preventing HIV infection in that country. It was nevertheless instructive to find that many of the issues raised by the Chinese had immediate parallels in my experience of the epidemic in the United States. Some of these issues belong to the nature of communicable disease. Some of them, however, belong to the cultural context of the disease, and I found in this regard less comforting parallels.

Most of the students knew that Magic Johnson—"a very famous American basketball player"—had announced his HIV diagnosis less than two months before my arrival. They also knew that infection and protection from infection did not depend on fame, class, or sexual orientation. But I sometimes wondered in speaking with these health professionals whether they recognized their own society's vulnerabilities to the epidemic. One physician who had spent a certain amount of time studying in California told me she did not think AIDS would be very much of a problem in China because, as she said, "The family situation is so strong in China." By this remark I understood her to mean that monogamous heterosexual marriage is a formidable bulwark against HIV infection. Certainly, that has been the message here in the United States from those who think that not only are moral ideals the pathway out of the epidemic but that the epidemic is the consequence of betrayal of those ideals. This same woman also noted that most Chinese do not have the money to bring them into contact with foreigners who would carry HIV infection, either by way of travel abroad or interaction with tourists traveling in China. "They do not have the money to go to the hotels here," she said.

Yet experience in the United States has shown that a social ideal of monogamous marriage has not proved a barrier to HIV infection in husband, wife, or children. And our experience here has shown too that lack of money—poverty especially—can prove a fertile ground for HIV infection rather than a barrier to it. While widespread HIV disease does not appear to be immediately likely in China, the American experience has shown that the belief in social immunity to HIV/AIDS may be in some respects an invitation to it. The history of the epidemic in the United States and around the world gives us reason enough to believe that *any* occurrence of AIDS is a disaster and not a problem to be ignored merely because it has not yet affected sufficient numbers of people or because the people it affects are not worthy of widespread social interest and concern. The course of the epidemic in the United States has shown the problems that ensue in attending to HIV/AIDS only when it appears to "seep out" of the marginalized classes in which it first appears.[21]

Given the example of the *China Daily* account that represented HIV/AIDS as a condition coming from abroad, from drug-users and prostitutes, the stage in China may be set to battle the epidemic on moral grounds; some of the attitudes I encountered suggest that some Chinese consider a certain set of moral ideals capable of preventing infection. The matter of homosexuality can be mentioned as an example. Certain features of China's accommodation of people's homoerotic interests may also prove an impediment—as happened elsewhere—to the iden-tification and control of HIV/AIDS. For most of its long history same-sex relations in China never became morally problematic as in Western European culture. On the contrary, there have been celebrated same-sex relations throughout Chinese history. Certain elements of the country's historical and political development, however, have led contemporary

China to a position officially critical of homoeroticism. In his *Passions of the Cut Sleeve* historian Bret Hinsch observes:

Many Chinese now regard the West as a cesspool of sexual and moral decadence. Outstripped by the West in material terms, they take consolation in their own ethical superiority. Chinese moralists often single out the recently imported "fad" of homosexuality as evidence of the spiritual pollution that now infects its place of origin—the United States and Europe. The Western vision of the decadent Orient is not matched with a parallel Chinese view of the exotic and depraved Occident. Yet ironically, the intolerance of homosexuality of which the Chinese are so proud actually originated in the West, while the acceptance of homosexuality that they abhor is more typical of native sexual ideals.[22]

I am not suggesting that HIV risk belongs even primarily to homosexuality in China, but moral and medical misunderstandings and intolerance of homosexuality make it more difficult to identify, address, and overcome any HIV infection that occurs through homosexual relations. A heterosexist culture can, as the Western experience shows, slow attention to the emergence of an epidemic and stall adequate educational efforts even when the epidemic is recognized and acknowledged. As in many aspects of China's culture, there are official and unofficial policies. While there may officially be no recognition of same-sex relations in that country, there are nevertheless persons who lead homoerotic lives, though success in such a life is often dependent on social privilege.[23] The challenge of meeting the future of homosexual HIV infection may therefore be impeded by "official" moral policies.

Even given an understanding of the epidemic, personal and cultural expectations can skew perceptions of educational messages. Talking with students on the last day of class, I found that a number of them had read the Gran Fury poster described above to mean that kissing *could* cause infection, even though these same students also fully understood that the activist goal of the poster was to challenge social inaction. Two physicians expressed concern about what a serious problem this form of transmission posed. (Such a construal may have also played a role in their thinking about what recommendations would be appropriate for health care workers with HIV.) My effort to correct the impression that kissing could cause HIV infection was met with skepticism. I even told one physician from a rural province that I myself had kissed people with HIV. "Why would you kiss someone with AIDS?" he asked, shocked, shaking his head as much in warning as disbelief. I responded that by every account with which I was familiar, kissing had not been demonstrated as a means of HIV infection. Against his exposure to ideas about the transmission of HIV, its links with immorality, and its lethal nature, I don't know that he was convinced. The expectation that HIV is highly communicable may be a cultural perception difficult to extinguish as people think about appropriate educational, policy, and punitive measures necessary to control the epidemic.

The important questions of AIDS education and prevention in China really are not different from the relevant questions elsewhere. Perhaps one of the most important is whether conceptual obstacles exist to prevent people from appreciating the significance of HIV and educating themselves against it. It may be that in China the perception that HIV is an exotic epidemic—in distant places, in homosexuals who have no place in China, in prostitutes who are morally avoidable persons, and in drug-users—may have the effect of impeding educational efforts, as such perceptions have elsewhere. Certainly China has advantages in a fight against HIV that the United States, for example, does not have. The government provision of health care means that the Chinese will not face certain of the difficulties often faced by PWAs in the United States. But it is worth wondering whether and to what extent those advantages may not be offset by other disadvantages in that culture's approaches to the epidemic.

These cultural concerns are not limited to China; they apply even to the United States today as it wrestles with sex surveys and condom advertisements. I wonder then whether each nation must find its own way in imagining and carrying forward an anti-AIDS program, whether in fact each country must stumble along on its own, unable to borrow clear lessons from other countries. To what extent will other countries—those at present largely unaffected by HIV—be able to avoid replicating certain of the problems like inattention, avoidance, marginalization, and substandard care faced in the United States. At a 1991 Beijing forum recognizing World AIDS Day, one far-sighted health official was quoted as saying that because the epidemic is still in its infancy there, China has an almost unique opportunity to prevent the spread of AIDS. He expressed hope that China would succeed in its fight against AIDS.[24]

There are many reasons to share such a hope, but some factors temper that hope as well. As the most populous nation on the planet, China occupies an unparalleled position in the world. It is true that the occurrence of HIV/AIDS in China has been so far slight, but given the way that *USA Today,* Cable Network News, and even robbery of taxi drivers at gunpoint have come to China, it is hard to imagine that HIV can be anything but a growing problem in that country. Perhaps if there is one lesson to be learned from experience around the globe, it is that to wait for large numbers of persons affected by HIV/AIDS before addressing the problem of the epidemic is to wait too long. From my experience I can say that Chinese people with fine minds are already capable of good dialogue about what policies ought to be adopted in order to prevent HIV infection. But in some respects Chinese society will have to be rethought—as U.S. society has had to be rethought—in order to find generally effective ways to help people protect themselves from infection. This rethinking would be a serious challenge for any country, but it may prove especially challenging for a country already struggling toward social development on so many fronts. I do hope that what efforts are adopted in China can avoid the fear-mongering, homophobia, and moral condemnation that to this day mar progress against AIDS in the United States, that the Chinese can avoid mistakes that even to this day take their toll in human disease and social opprobrium. In this regard maybe a good place to start AIDS education in China as elsewhere would be with explanations that kissing doesn't kill.

PART THREE

AIDS Politics

8

HIV at the Borders

In 1987 Senator Jesse Helms sponsored a bill subsequently approved by Congress that added AIDS to the medical conditions barring the entry of affected foreign nationals into the United States.[1] This ban was supported by some health professions organizations worried about the public health of the nation and the costs of publicly supported care for people with AIDS.[2] The entry of "foreigners" into the United States has long been a concern to its "natives." Indeed, the history of exclusion from the U.S. has often had as its goal the barring of persons judged religiously, ideologically, racially, or economically harmful to the country. It was the efforts to bar the Chinese "yellow peril" which in 1882 prompted the first federal legislation establishing limitations on immigration. A nation of immigrants, the U.S. has nevertheless sought to exercise considerable control over who does and does not enter the country. Medical conditions that have in the past been used to exclude foreign nationals from the United States include a long list of human debilitations. One 1934 report on conditions at Ellis Island blithely listed those who must be excluded by law thus: "idiots, imbeciles, feeble-minded persons, epileptics, insane persons who have had one or more attacks of insanity previously, persons of psychopathic constitutional inferiority, persons afflicted with a loath[e]some or dangerous contagious condition, including venereal disease, trachoma, and certain chronic conditions."[3]

The exclusion of foreign nationals with HIV thus continued a history that careens between the nation's moral commitment to ideals of equality and social justice and the ideological, economic, and health factors that strain willingness to admit all who wish to enter the country. The United States has traditionally represented itself as an asylum open to refugees. Emma Lazarus's words inscribed on the Statue of Liberty bespeak a vaunted welcome to the dispossessed: "Give me your tired, your poor, / Your huddled masses yearning to breathe free, / The wretched refuse of your teeming shore, / Send these, the homeless, tempest-tossed to me: / I lift my lamp beside the golden door." Yet nativist movements interested in racial and political purity as well as economic organizations worried about job competition have often sought stringent exclusion of foreign nationals. The bar to foreign nationals with HIV continues a debate that has for hundreds of years engaged "natives" about the worth and admissibility of "foreigners."

Although Helms's 1987 proposal gained congressional approval, the bar on entry of persons with HIV drew criticism from a number of leading AIDS policy analysts around the world. The exclusionary policy put the United States not in the company of progressive, developed nations but in the company of nations less well regarded for their policies on human rights. June Osborn of the National Commission on AIDS said the policy of excluding people with HIV was counterproductive, discriminatory, and a waste of resources.[4] More important, she thought, the bar suggests that HIV infection is easily communicated. In fact, the ban was later modified to limit exclusion to persons seeking permanent residence in the U.S. and to permit temporary entry to others under limited conditions.[5] During his 1992 presidential campaign Bill Clinton announced himself as opposed to even this form of the ban. Following his election, however, he let the policy stand, and Congress acted to formalize the administrative policy in law.[6] We must now ask whether arguments used to defend the exclusion of foreign nationals with HIV (except under the limited circumstances of the current policy) are convincing. I suggest that the exclusionary policy is not in fact justified in the name of protecting the public health, that its justification in terms of economic costs is unconvincing because the policy is selective in what it deems unacceptably costly, and that the costs are not as disproportionately high as they have been represented in the debate. Far from protecting the common good or protecting the nation's health costs, the policy draws on the worst xenophobic traditions of the United States.

Closing the Door

Because the original bar on all foreign nationals with HIV was criticized and deemed excessively exclusionary, modifications of the policy permitted the limited entry of foreign nationals who declare their condition and who enter the country only temporarily and for a specified purpose.[7] This modified policy remains controversial for a number of reasons. The 1990 Immigration Act redefined the medical exclusions in such a way as to bar persons only if they had a communicable disease of public health significance.[8] The CDC in February 1990 recommended that AIDS and all other communicable diseases except infectious tuberculosis be removed from the list of diseases that bar entry into the United States.[9] In January 1991 then-U.S. Secretary for the Department of Health and Human Services (DHHS) Louis W. Sullivan proposed not only removing HIV infection from the list but retaining only infectious tuberculosis as the sole disease on that list. In defense of his proposal Sullivan said that AIDS was not spread through casual contact but through sexual intercourse and contaminated needles. As required by law, Sullivan offered the public a period of comment before allowing the policy to take effect.

Comment on the proposal was not long in coming, especially from conservative quarters. Influential in this regard was a torrent of letters, as many as forty thousand, received by various government agencies, protesting the proposed change. One anonymous health department official characterized the letters as expressing fear of inundating the medical care system with the care of PWAs and objecting to any increased taxes necessary to pay for that care. The same official said he believed that many of the letters were prompted by an evangelical broadcaster's appeal to write, since the letters were often similar in content.[10]

Sullivan's proposed change also set off a squabble within federal agencies. The Department of Justice, which has jurisdiction over the Immigration and Naturalization Service (INS), objected to Sullivan's proposal for a number of reasons, saying that it had not been adequately consulted and that it did not believe that Sullivan's view that AIDS was not a disease of public health significance had been adequately documented.[11] President George Bush himself came to the defense of the exclusionary policy. Federal health officials reiterated that a specific HIV bar was unnecessary because HIV infection was not casually transmitted and explained that if cost was the issue, then the INS already had authority to bar the entry of any persons who were likely to become a costly public charge. The Justice Department rejected this view, saying that it was impracticable when admitting persons to the U.S. to require the sophisticated medical and health coverage analysis that would enable them to determine who was likely to become such a public charge.[12]

Because of the controversy surrounding the proposal to remove HIV from the list of medical exclusions, the policy was continued beyond its original expiration date.[13] In the end the policy was not changed, and persons with HIV are barred from permanent residence in this country and may visit temporarily only with special permission. Persons entering the U.S. are expected to declare their HIV infection and obtain appropriate permission to enter. A *New York Times* editorial lampooned the policy: "Its chief effect is to make the United States a laughing stock in world medical circles. This policy should be abandoned quickly."[14] Harvey V. Fineberg, dean of Harvard's School of Public Health, said of continuing the policy: "The result would be the continuing, needless humiliation of travelers, a blow to international cooperation in the struggle against AIDS, a distraction from the real sources of infection at home, and not one iota of added protection of the public." He added: "The real reasons behind the exclusionary policy are unstated—irrational fear, misunderstanding and prejudice, salted by political opportunism and cowardice. Foreigners make an easy target, especially those with a dread disease associated with a lifestyle some despise. Excluding those with HIV infection is a surrogate for keeping out social undesirables."[15] In protest of the policy the organizers of the Eighth International Conference on AIDS canceled Boston as the 1992 conference site and moved the meeting to Amsterdam.[16] Organizers said they could not guarantee admittance of attendees to the country, although since PWAs are theoretically permitted to enter the U.S. temporarily, protest rather than visa worries no doubt motivated this decision.

When asked about the cancellation of the Boston site, President George Bush said it was "too bad" but he expressed optimism: "They'll find other ways of getting together, so it doesn't bother me." Asked if he was reconsidering the policy, Bush said, "That policy is a good, sound policy. The American people, I think, are supportive of it."[17] Former U.S. Representative William E. Dannemeyer also favored continuance of the bar: "I'm very pleased that [D]HHS woke up to the absurdity of this proposal [to modify the exclusionary list], and I hope it stays buried in the bottom of a circular file in the deepest innards of the bureaucracy.... It was ludicrous what they were saying. On the one hand they say AIDS is a major problem; on the other hand they say we should take in HIV carriers with impunity."[18] Dannemeyer had of course been the sponsor of a number of highly restrictive AIDS proposals. His book *Shadow in the Land* describes the many evils of AIDS and the ways he alleges AIDS efforts serve as a front for prohomosexual ideology.[19] Dannemeyer believes in the immorality of homoeroticism and sees AIDS as its inevitable consequence. The associations of AIDS with immorality have been a feature of discourse about the epidemic since the very beginning.[20] And yet the arguments advanced in favor of the exclusionary policy were not conducted primarily in the language of morals. They were conducted in the language of protecting the public health and protecting the health-care system. Are the arguments as value-free as terminology of this kind might suggest?

Protecting the Public Health

Will the current entry policy protect the public health of the United States? Is it this policy, alone or in conjunction with other national efforts, an important part of an anti-AIDS program?

In May 1991 the DHHS estimated the expected number of HIV-positive persons who might be admitted to the United States each year at 600 to 800 persons. In 1989 420 would-be immigrants were barred after an HIV infection was uncovered.[21] Canadian law and medicine professor Margaret Somerville noted that the 1989 modifications to the original exclusionary policy of 1987 allowed entry to the United States by foreign nationals if they established:

that their entry into the United States would confer a public health benefit which outweighs any risk to the public health. A sufficient public benefit can include showing that the short term non-immigrant will be attending academic or health related activities (including seeking medical treatment), or conducting temporary business in the U.S. A sufficient public benefit can also include the applicant establishing that he or she will visit close family members in the United States. Entry into the United States essentially for tourism reasons alone does not constitute the requisite benefit to overcome the risk.[22]

This policy in many ways carries with it the kinds of moralistic views of AIDS that have prevailed in the United States since 1981. Foreign nationals may be admitted to the country provided they are here for *serious* purposes like family visitation and commerce, that is, sufficiently sexless and drug-free activities incompatible with risk of infection to citizens. A government need not be worried about family visitation and business as predatory, and neither do family visitation or commerce tempt a weak-willed population to succumb to the temptations of "imported" sex and needles. By contrast, "tourism" follows the pathways of the pleasure principle and is therefore judged antagonistic to the public health. Given a deeply embedded cultural view of the AIDS epidemic as emerging from sexual and narcotic hedonism, it is tempting to see the *Guide Michelin* or, better, the gay *Bob Damron's Address Book* as the guidebook public health officials ought to use in tracking down and controlling the epidemic.

Of course, the central question is not whether business is more or less "moral" than tourism but whether the entry of foreign nationals with HIV represents a significant risk of new infection in the United States. Over a third of a million cases of AIDS have already been diagnosed in this country. It is estimated that there may be as many as one million more cases of HIV infection. Contrasted with such numbers, the number of foreign nationals with HIV could represent only a tiny fraction of the total number of HIV/AIDS diagnoses in the country. Moreover, is the entry of infected foreign nationals a significant addition to the annual number of new HIV/AIDS cases when compared to the number of new infections that occur through sexual intercourse or needle-sharing in this country? The United States has the highest prevalence of HIV of any developed country. Even the addition of the DHSS's maximum estimate of eight hundred persons with HIV/AIDS per year would not appear to significantly affect either the incidence or prevalence of HIV/AIDS in this country.

That the United States has so many people with HIV is significant when considered in light of what the country has not chosen to do with respect to its own citizens' travel. The U.S. does not bar its citizens with HIV from leaving the country. So by its exclusionary policy the U.S. asserts a duty it does not itself honor: keeping citizens with HIV at home.[23] Foreign nationals with HIV may not ordinarily visit this country for purposes of tourism. But any U.S. citizen with HIV may travel abroad for such a reason and, to use Dannemeyer's language, do so "with impunity." (Such visitors may, of course, find barriers to travel in a few countries, but even those barriers are not so stringent that they cannot be evaded.) The U.S. does not recognize any parallel between reasons for keeping foreign nationals with HIV out and reasons for keeping citizens with HIV at home. An ironic effect might be the future exclusion of a legitimate visitor to the U.S. who contracted an HIV infection from *an American* while here.[24] Clearly, current policy does more to hold foreign nationals in contempt than it does to prevent new HIV infections.

The bar on entry to foreign nationals with HIV/AIDS can also be read as a public health failure if the American population must be defended through prophylactic measures at the border. If Americans are not educated or prepared to protect themselves individually from HIV infection in their sexual and needle-using habits, then it is understandable that they would want immigration officials policing the borders. The very desirability of such a policy indicates that people are unable or unwilling to assume responsibility for protecting themselves from HIV infection. A population capable of practicing safe sex and safe needle use would not need the protection of immigration officials. It would be unfortunate if support for an exclusionary policy calibrated the extent to which Americans feel unable to protect themselves from HIV risk and look to statist efforts to lift the burden from them. Or, worse, the bar on entry to foreign nationals with HIV may represent the way persons not (yet) affected by the epidemic calculate its significance: not in terms of the swath of sickness and death it has cut across this nation but in terms of its imagined economic costs in future tax-supported health care.

Protecting the Taxpayer

Those who recognize the limitations of defending the exclusionary bar as protection of the public's health may justify the bar as a matter of protecting the taxpayer's wallet. This justification is now the one most often used in defense of the policy. The high costs of treating PWAs has been from the beginning of the epidemic the subject of extensive media coverage and economic analysis. The costs can be in fact quite formidable. One U.S. senator, for example, has said, "I do not think it is compassionate to open up a sign that says: 'Come to America and Uncle Sam is going to take care of your medical expenses.'"[25]

The arguments in favor of excluding foreign nationals with HIV typically fail to take into account two factors that influence the economic costs of immigrants. Margaret Somerville has pointed out in her discussion of immigration policies in Canada that while groups of immigrants and refugees generally do increase demands on public services such individuals also offset those costs through their employment or other contributions to the economy including increased demand for consumer goods.[26] We need to keep in mind that health-care services too contribute to employment in significant ways. In addition, it is unclear that admission of foreign nationals with HIV would necessarily prove more costly than the admission of other people needing expensive health treatments for cancer, kidney, and heart disease.[27] The government does not attempt to identify and exclude *any other class* of individuals by reason of health-care costs they might create. Moreover, this focus on the (excessive) health costs that foreign nationals with HIV might create in the United States serves to obscure an underlying assumption about the U.S. health-care system. To argue that foreign nationals would overburden the system implies that the health-care system is at present adequately designed. This view is highly questionable in light of the general consensus that large numbers of Americans already fail to receive adequate health-care; moreover, cross-cultural comparisons that assess general measures of morbidity and mortality cast U.S. health care in a poor light in cost of services relative to benefit. Indeed, we may wonder whether worry about the overburdening of the health-care system is not more a generalized worry about the fragile state of the system at present than a specific worry that it will be overwhelmed by foreign nationals with HIV. In any case, the focus on costs of foreign nationals with HIV also suggests that patients must be suitable for the health-care system rather than the opposite.

In an editorial urging a rescinding of the ban the *New York Times* quickly dismissed the ban on temporary visitors as "silly." The editors, however, express sympathy with the concern about the cost of foreign nationals with HIV in the country for extended periods of time, admitting that the longer foreigners stay in the U.S. "the greater the chance some might spread the virus or require care." The editorial continues, using the government's statistics against the policy: "By one government estimate, only about six hundred AIDS-infected individuals would be admitted as permanent residents each year—compared with one million Americans already infected. And finding them among the six hundred thousand admitted each year would require costly testing. If the goal is to fight AIDS, this is not where to spend the money."[28] While the editorial does hesitate about the question of permanent residents and naturalized citizens with HIV, it nonetheless recognizes that in the long run the question of foreign nationals is relatively unimportant. But even this view too easily presumes a compelling economic argument. It is hard to give credence to the view that people with HIV are lined up at American consulates around the world in order to be permitted the luxury of treatment and care at Boston City Hospital or Cook County Hospital or any of the other public health-care institutions in the United States. If people are motivated to come to the United States, one must assume that they seek a general rise in their overall standard of living; it would certainly not make good sense for foreign nationals to pursue help from one of the least accessible health-care systems in the world. And in any case, those many thousands of foreign nationals already in the United States illegally—by overextending visa permissions or simply entering without inspection—do not have legal access to many publicly funded health-care resources. Certain classes of foreign nationals do tend to use public resources at rates higher than others, but they do not do so in any uniform way.[29] Even if all HIV-infected foreign nationals needed health care, we cannot assume that they would all generate the same costs or be equally dependent on the U.S. taxpayer. It is not even clear that the figures that are typically bandied about in the debate reflect accurately on the costs of PWAs. Though one study did report an approximate cost of $147,000 for medical care from diagnosis to death for a PWA, more recent studies put the direct lifetime medical costs between $40,000 and $50,000, making AIDS comparable in cost to some conditions and less costly than others that foreign nationals might have.[30]

The question of public health and health-care costs becomes academic here inasmuch as the exclusionary ban cannot be expected to prevent the entry of every foreign national with HIV. The solution to the endangerment of the American public from HIV lies in enabling the American public to protect itself, each person individually. The solution to the burdens imposed on the health-care system by persons with HIV, foreign nationals or not, is a restructuring of the health-care system, one of the very topics-in-chief during the 1992 presidential election. Perhaps the notion that HIV infection is an avoidable risk (if only one avoids certain sexual and drug-using practices) also fuels the notion that infected foreign nationals are unworthy of admission to the United States and access to its health-care institutions. That no objections are raised to health costs incurred by foreign nationals with cancer or heart disease, which can also have their basis in personal choices, suggests that the economic argument is only an epiphenomenal manifestation of deeper social mistrust of people with HIV. Such mistrust is not novel in U.S. history. The mistrust of certain classes of people has historically expressed itself through exclusion on the basis of medical diagnoses, as if social problems could be remedied through the exclusion of certain diseases.[31] Certain diseases such as syphilis were taken as a synecdoche for the entire moral and civic merit of a person. In order to achieve certain political and moral ends, such mistrust literalizes the notion of the body politic in order to menace it with sickness and death. The xenophobia behind such views is worth considering in detail.

HIV Xenophobia

The barrier to foreign nationals with HIV should be interpreted against the emergence of AIDS in this country, especially as that involved Haitians. Early in the 1980s Haitians residing in the United States appeared to be affected disproportionately by AIDS. Later, however, critics blamed this identification on cultural insensitivity that blurred the vision of epidemiologists looking for causes of AIDS. The focus on Haitians, critics said, resulted from (*a*) a lack of appreciation of the reluctance of Haitians to admit to behaviors perceived as leading to deportation, (*b*) an insensitivity to the question of homoeroticism in men of that culture, (*c*) an enthusiasm for associating AIDS with the lore surrounding voodoo, and, perhaps as general context, (*d*) a disposition to single out for selective treatment the impoverished black inhabitants of the Western Hemisphere's poorest country.[32] In previous times, syphilis, not AIDS, had been called the disease of Haiti.[33]

Haitians to this day continue to challenge U.S. AIDS policy. Haitians fleeing their native country have created a policy dilemma regarding their treatment as refugees. Because of current policy, all persons entering the U.S., even refugees, must declare their HIV infection. At a camp at the Guantánamo naval base in Cuba, the United States held for a time more than two hundred Haitian refugees with HIV infections, refugees whose goal was permanent relocation to the United States. One associate deputy attorney general admitted that the Justice Department would just as soon have looked the other way on the HIV exclusion policy. Ironically, though, it was the Justice Department itself that resisted the DHHS proposal to remove the HIV bar. In frustration over the identification and detainment of Haitians with HIV, that same Justice Department official said "that it was now clear that the easiest thing to have done would have been to avoid testing the immigrants for HIV and simply treat their claims as those of other Haitians who must prove under immigration law that they fear political persecution in order to be granted asylum in the United States." He did add that while everyone involved in the case thought it would have been simpler not to test for HIV, "no one in the Administration was comfortable with remaining ignorant."[34] The same Republican administration that in good conscience could neither admit these detainees nor repatriate them involuntarily did have, however, the luxury of passing their Haitian problem on to the next president, who had said while campaigning that he would lift the ban on immigrants infected with HIV. During the transition to the new administration, however, Bill Clinton reaffirmed the previous administration's policy of turning back Haitians who approached the U.S., arguing that such a decision was necessary to protect them from the dangers of their unseaworthy ships.[35] Since the 1993 presidential inauguration the U.S. Congress has acted to affirm as federal statute the bar on immigration by persons with HIV.[36] Ironically, not long afterward a federal U.S. court ordered the immediate release of the people being held in Guantánamo, and they were brought to this country.[37] The Clinton administration let that event go forward without any immediate appeal though legal challenges remain possible.

The U.S. exclusionary policy simply reverses the logic of quarantine. Rather than exiling people with HIV, the United States has put itself into quarantine against the exogenous masses with HIV. Fear of strangers may constitute part of the motive for the bar, but exclusion also taps deeply into the national psyche about who is and who is not fit to visit, let alone become a resident or citizen of, the United States. The original enactment of the exclusionary policy in 1987 may have followed increased public fear about the epidemic and its control, especially given the way the epidemic catapulted to media prominence in 1986 and 1987. Yet the reaffirmation of the policy in 1992 may reflect not only that original fear but also despair that despite all the headlines reporting progress biomedicine has nevertheless failed to offer either a cure for or vaccine against HIV infection.

Margaret Somerville has pointed out that legislators may be inclined to single out immigrants for restriction because immigrants and refugees lack political clout. Such restrictions offer evidence that legislators are willing to do something about AIDS but only if they can avoid alienating any constituency.[38] Given the fear of the epidemic and biomedicine's failure to contain it, the exclusionary bar offers certain moral and political assurance that the nation is doing something to protect its citizens, an assurance that feeds a public hungry for certainty in the midst of an ever-growing epidemic and a public wary of the emergence of gay men, condoms, safe-sex talk, and needle-cleaning bleach kits into plain view. The exclusionary policy can thus assuage anxiety by distancing the epidemic from the American population and by asserting a territorial limit to its advances. The bar is the medical equivalent of the twelve-mile border zone that protects the nation's shores. The bar strategically relieves Americans of part of the responsibility for the protection of their own health inasmuch as the visitors who would endanger them are presumably policed at the borders: anybody who gets through should be "clean."

In many ways exclusion is merely the continuation of old policies through new language. For example, certain nativist opposition to immigration has expressed itself in the association of drugs with certain populations around the world: hashish, African; opium, Asian; cocaine, South American; heroin, European. The ills associated with drugs were interpreted as racial weaknesses justifying hostile immigration policies.[39] The association of HIV infection with drug use then reenacts certain nativist hostilities to foreigners. The association of HIV infection with gay men also reenacts historical hostilities. Until recently the exclusion of homosexual men and women from the United States was permitted under certain immigration laws barring the entry of "undesirable" persons.[40] Together, the exclusion of persons with HIV recasts the historical exclusion of drug-users and gay men (and lesbians) in terms of their infectiousness and cost rather than their alleged psychopathic personalities and unwanted political views.

The Wretched Refuse of Your Teeming Shore

The problem of foreign nationals with HIV is not really about the people with HIV who would in fact come to the United States. The problem is the perception of those who *could* come. An open-door policy raises the specter of the millions of people with HIV abroad who *could conceivably* come to the U.S. Given the reports of AIDS rampant in Africa, for example, mere eligibility alone is threatening. Mere eligibility over-shadows realistic assessment of the actual numbers of persons who in fact seek entrance. Thus construed, the question of people with HIV in-fection invokes and continues the fear of the teeming, wretched masses that inspired earlier xenophobia. It is these perceived teeming masses—not the actual 420 would-be immigrants who applied in 1989—who in the public imagination threaten the public health and who tax the public coffers. As the notion of entry to this country is deeply tied to the notion of privilege,[41] we should not be surprised that certain qualifications are demanded of immigrants by the native, nativist population. People with HIV are not perceived as immigrants who will add to the social or political advance of the country. They are seen as offering nothing but their economic need and their infectious selves.

It is unlikely that an exclusionary policy will succeed in protecting the nation against widespread prevalence of HIV any more than isolation theories rooted in bacteriology or other theories of disease did before it. The exclusionary policy functionally narrows the focus of anti-HIV efforts at the expense of efforts aimed at social and environmental influences.[42] As Harvey V. Fineberg has noted, the bar will certainly extend cultural judgments about who is and who is not worthy to enter the United States. The mission of the policy is to keep out, as he says, "social undesirables."[43] In particular, the bar works to exclude gay men and drug-users. Foreign nationals with HIV who are not gay men or drug-users nevertheless *function* as gay men and drug-users inasmuch as they undermine the cultural divide that putatively exists between the infected and uninfected, the "straight" and the "not straight." Insofar as foreign nationals with HIV are "straight," they betray their own kind for they, not gay men and drug-users, imperil the native heterosexuals and non-drug-users. Their potential for infection is therefore especially to be feared. The exclusionary bar therefore underlines the perception that the "straight" in either a sexual or narcotic sense do not have HIV.

AIDS activists have long noted the effort of government to distance itself from the epidemic. The absence of strong presidential leadership on AIDS during its first decade and the ban on funding of educational materials that might conceivably "promote" homosexuality or drug use are both examples of the failure of government to assume a role in combatting the epidemic. The government's advocacy of the view[44] and the U.S. Supreme Court's eventual concurrence that employers can retroactively limit health-care coverage in employees with AIDS is an-other example of the government's banishing of the epidemic to the margins of social concern.[45] The denial of entry of foreign nationals into the United States belongs alongside these examples because the bar officially weakens as a matter of government policy any responsibility to people with HIV and amounts to the politically easiest and least reliable means of fighting the epidemic among its citizens. The policy, in fact, suggests that American public morality and citizenship are intimately bound up with the notion of health. Past exclusionary efforts declared whole classes of people unfit to serve the nation in its moral and political ideals. Irish immigrants, for example, were thought to be unfit for the rigors of free citizenship by reason of their Roman Catholicism, which religion allegedly made them dependent on ecclesiastical authority.[46] Foreign nationals with HIV, by contrast, are seen as unfit for citizenship by reason of their immunological impairment, which makes them dependent on the health-care system.

Ironically, the United States has often championed the right of emigration, for example, the right of Jews to emigrate from the USSR.[47] It has championed a right whose corresponding duty—the duty to take in emigrants—it disavows as applied to people with HIV. There are many legitimate reasons why a nation may bar certain visitors and immigrants, but the bar on entry of people with HIV is morally questionable because it appears to be a matter of selective enforcement unjustified even according to the arguments by which it is advanced. If individual Americans were capable of protecting themselves against HIV risk, then the presence of foreign nationals with HIV could not endanger them. Moreover, visitation and immigration policies cannot significantly alter the incidence or prevalence of HIV disease and hence overall national health costs. And even if the costs of health care in the nation were increased, the singling out of the HIV syndrome for exclusionary treatment is unjust when foreign nationals with other potentially costly diseases are ignored. Against such a background the HIV exclusionary bar reveals itself as an exercise in the xenophobic logic one finds elsewhere in the history of United States immigration policy. Immigrants and refugees have in the past been judged unfit for entry by reason of race, religion, and health. Like the ignominy of American slavery contrasted with the early republic's declarations of universal human equality, such exclusion continues to mock the professed ideals of this nation.

The embrace of interdiction as an easy solution to the epidemic, however, is likely to prove no more effective than immigrant literacy tests in the early part of this century[48] in keeping away the unwanted. Given the many ways in which the exclusionary policy is evadable and given the ways in which it can only be selectively enforced, such a bar functions less as an actual prophylactic barrier to new infections in Americans or as a cost-control measure protecting the nation's health-care system from overload than as a merging of xenophobic and homophobic attitudes offered in the name of an *idealized* American population. National and personal identity exist in part only by defining themselves against something else, preferably something less worthy so as also to permit the assertion of moral superiority.[49] The exclusionary policy is as much an assertion of identity as an act of public health and fiscal responsibility. But other ways to conceive national identity exist. The nation might set aside the exclusionary bar and lift the lamp that in the past has served it so well. Since record-keeping began, the U.S. has absorbed more than fifty million legal immigrants from at least a hundred and fifty foreign countries.[50] As it has in the past, this nation may yet find a way to prove in the case of people with HIV that it can be indeed the refuge of the dispossessed.

9

Politics and Priorities

The standing of the AIDS epidemic in U.S. political consciousness was evident by the role it came to occupy in the 1992 presidential election. By 1987 the presidential candidates of the major political parties had all discussed AIDS in public, although the subject did not assume a central status in the election.[1] By 1992, however, AIDS had became a matter requiring attention from political candidates; witness its discussion in the presidential debates of that year, where the issue took its place alongside the economy, the military, and abortion as matters of fundamental public interest. In the first presidential candidate debate, for example, George Bush, Ross Perot, and Bill Clinton all addressed various aspects of the epidemic.[2] Their remarks reveal the way these candidates viewed the epidemic and the position they accorded it in the nation's priorities. Their remarks are also worth juxtaposing to the conclusions of a 1993 report of a National Research Council panel on the social impact of AIDS. That report, which concluded that AIDS has failed to have an impact on major social institutions or directly affect most Americans, was received with concern by AIDS activists who believed that its conclusions justified inattention and insensitivity to the continuing tragedy of the epidemic. Nevertheless, the report and the remarks of the presidential candidates offer an understanding of the obligations a society has in regard to research, treatment, and prevention in the epidemic. These views are important cultural artifacts that reflect how AIDS is understood as a moral priority in the nation's goals.

The Republican Candidate

The topic of AIDS was introduced by a member of the panel of journalists whose questions structured the first 1992 presidential "debate." Although candidates' responses during the forum were constrained by time, format, and election strategy, their remarks there indicate their conception of the responsibility of government in the epidemic. The question about AIDS was directed to George Bush, with the understanding that Ross Perot and Bill Clinton would also have time to respond: "Mr. President, yesterday tens of thousands of people paraded past the White House to demonstrate their concern abut the disease AIDS; a celebrated member of your commission, Magic Johnson, quit, saying that there was too much inaction. Where is this widespread feeling coming from that your Administration is not doing enough about AIDS?"[3] President Bush spoke at greater length than the other two candidates:

It's coming from the political process. We have increased funding on AIDS, we've doubled it, on research and on every other aspect. My request for this year was $4.9 billion for AIDS, ten times as much per AIDS victim as per cancer victim.

I think we're showing the proper compassion and concern, so I can't tell you where it's coming from, but I am very much concerned about AIDS and I believe that we've got the best researchers in the world out there at NIH working the problem. We're funding them. I wish there was more money, but we're funding them far more than any time in the past, and we're going to keep on doing that.

I don't know. I was a little disappointed in Magic because he came to me and I said, "Now, if you see something we're not doing, get a hold of me, call me, let me know." He went to one meeting, and then we heard that he was stepping down. So he's been replaced by Mary Fisher, who electrified the Republican convention by talking about the compassion and the concern that we feel. It was a beautiful moment and I think she'll do a first-class job on that commission.

It is, of course, a standard rhetorical tactic in politics to suggest as Bush did that public dissatisfaction with a given administration's policy on any topic is the result of antagonism generated by the opposition. This allegation is, however, buttressed by Bush's subsequent explanation that outlined a program centering AIDS at the heart of a nationally coordinated effort supported by the best researchers with more money at their disposal than is available for any other biomedical effort. Despite the significant measures already under way, Bush nevertheless expressed regret that he could not do more, signaling that his intentions in this regard are constrained by the limits of federal government. He did vow to continue funding NIH researchers in significant ways following his reelection.

Bush treated the question of Johnson's resignation from the AIDS commission as regrettable, but the president shifted blame away from himself. Bush maintained that he had made it clear that Johnson had access to him and that he expected Johnson's help in making suggestions. As Johnson's replacement, Bush proposed Mary Fisher, who is said to be qualified for the commission because of her ability to express the compassion and concern that "we" feel.[4]

In an apparent attempt to score points against Bill Clinton, Bush then wandered off the topic of AIDS (these discussions are not quoted here) with some remarks about civil rights legislation, discrimination, and a denial of Ross Perot's contention that "we" don't have the will to fight drugs. Bush returned to the topic of AIDS by linking it with behavior:

And I once called on somebody, "Well, change your behavior; if the behavior you're using is prone to cause AIDS, change the behavior."
    Next thing I know, one of these ACT Up groups is out saying, "Bush ought to change *his* behavior." You can't talk about it rationally; the extremes are hurting the AIDS cause. To go into a Catholic mass, in a beautiful cathedral in New York, under the cause of helping in AIDS and start throwing condoms around in the mass, I'm sorry, I think it sets back the cause. We cannot move to the extreme. We've got to care, we've got to continue everything we can at the federal and the local level. Barbara, I think, is doing a superb job in destroying the myth about AIDS. And all of us are in this fight together, all of us care. Do not go to the extreme.
    So I think the appeal is, yes, we care. And the other thing is part of AIDS—it's [the sense] people cannot be brought together, we can't turn this country around. If we can come together, nothing, *nothing,* can stop us.

In many ways Bush's latter statements contain views that have pervaded discussion and silence about AIDS since the onset of the epidemic.

In discussing AIDS as comparable to issues of drug use, civil rights, and discrimination Bush situated AIDS as a problem outside the domain of biomedicine: AIDS is a problem that has its origins in individual behavior. Bush thus espoused the sentiment that if only people took more responsibility for their choices, if only they walked away from endangering behaviors, then AIDS could be controlled not by biomedical intervention but by attrition, by eliminating new cases of HIV infection. The implication of this view is that while the government is operating full-tilt in its biomedical research capacities, individuals are personally evading responsibility for avoidance of HIV infection. The guilty behavior implied but not enunciated by Bush includes unprotected sexual intercourse and shared needles. Bush's counsel thus becomes a variant of the "Just say no" tactics associated with Nancy Reagan's campaign against drug use.

Yet this kind of "solution" to the epidemic proposes a kind of personal responsibility that functions as an ideal little reflected in the sexual and drug lives of human beings. Certainly, espousing a "Just say no" policy reveals a great deal about the temptations a sexagenarian president does not face or even understand. That he finds the solution to AIDS in "just" changing behavior suggests that he cannot acknowledge the place of such risks as drug use and receptive anal intercourse in the lives of others. In addition, such a simplistic "solution" suggests that these risks are not only trivial but avoidable through a kind of common sense supposed to be sufficiently present across the breadth of American society.

Changing behavior, however, is a highly complex matter. Even where motivation is high, changes do not always follow human efforts. It is simply unknown, for example, what kind of educational efforts will enable a gay man to avoid risk behavior throughout his life or what knowledge will help a heterosexual, drug-using woman from putting others at risk of infection when she knows herself to be HIV-infected. We simply do not know what kind of psychosocial supports are necessary to help gay and straight teenagers grappling with drugs avoid centering their lives around drug culture and its HIV risks. Given human fallibility, is it fair to single out and blame people who incur an HIV infection any more than people who, for instance, court the dangers of a nutritionally impoverished diet? The accusation that HIV infection is self-incurred is not adequate justification for the general conclusion that people can protect themselves from HIV infection any more than people can protect themselves from the smoking or diet-related illness and death. This is certainly not to say that people shouldn't change their behavior where they can or that educational efforts should not be exerted toward this extremely important goal, but it is to say that human decisions are complex matters often intractable even to the best advice.

Bush's use of the term *victim*, of course, offends all sensibilities attuned to the victimizing effects of that word's connotations of passivity and helplessness. Though this point has been made repeatedly, the language of victimology continues to pervade public discussion about

AIDS. It is, though, more important to note that the way in which Bush framed the question of AIDS funding opened the door to invidious comparisons: Why is AIDS getting so much more money per "victim" if in fact people could avoid it? Why aren't people with other diseases getting more money for the study and treatment of the *involuntary* conditions that afflict so many? By framing the issue this way, Bush in effect undercut his own claim that he would like to do more for AIDS because in identifying the amount of money spent "on AIDS," he drew attention to the way in which other diseases were not equivalently funded. He set the stage for a consideration of whether AIDS isn't in fact preferentially treated, especially given its alleged avoidability. And if such was not the president's intention, then it may be interpreted another way: as suggesting that other diseases are *under*funded and that perhaps they should be better funded. Such an interpretation, though, is unlikely for a candidate who vowed—for a famous second time—no new taxes.

What Mr. Bush *did not* reveal during this debate was his own record. While he was vice-president under Ronald Reagan, Bush was chairman of the President's Task Force on Regulatory Relief, which recommended planning at the Food and Drug Administration (FDA) that led to greater accessibility of experimental drugs. He also recommended the creation of another committee to study and streamline new procedures for the approval of new drugs for AIDS and cancer.[5] While the role of AIDS activists in spurring federal interest in drug development and experimentation has certainly been a formidable one, the antiregulatory and antibureaucratic spirit brought to the federal government under Reagan and Bush administrations also contributed to the opening of experimental AIDS drugs to persons outside formal drug trials, even if the motives of government minimalists were quite different from those of AIDS activists. Perhaps Bush did not find time under the constraints of the debate to note his role, but he had in fact a certain claim to the status of AIDS activist.

But Bush had only harsh words for AIDS activists. His remarks on ACT UP label them extremists who are unable to talk about AIDS rationally. In this way he suspends any requirement to take their views and actions seriously; in his discourse they are figuratively and literally irrational and others are thereby better situated to formulate AIDS policies. This characterization of activists also invites psychological remedies for them, not political remedies for the epidemic. After labeling AIDS activists as irrational, he then paints them as political extremists by referring in a disappointed fashion to the 1989 disruption of a Roman Catholic mass at New York's St. Patrick's Cathedral, a confrontation that protested Catholic views of sexuality and AIDS education.[6] To raise the image of AIDS activists in violation of ecclesiastical sanctuary was to raise the specter of an uncontrollable political group in a way that would undercut sympathy for AIDS activists efforts. In sum, George Bush's depiction of AIDS activists recalls the characteristics of activists most likely to offend; he does not mention any of their efforts directed at health-care reform. Bush does not see ACT UP in the long tradition of American dissent and political reformism; he sees only extremism.[7] His final words on the topic of AIDS propose not the reform of any social attitudes or practices but the reform of AIDS activists themselves: "Do not go to the extreme." Do we have any reason to believe that "moderation" by itself will lead to control of the AIDS epidemic?

Bush's public remarks are often disjointed, even mangled, and the remarks he offered by way of answer to the original question are typical in this regard. He does emphasize that "we" care and that if united there is nothing that can stop "us." Who is "us," of course, is a question that preoccupied the 1992 Republican national convention speakers who stressed the divisions in American culture. In contrast to the rules of eligibility for "God's country" stressed at that convention, Bush's "us" here is an undifferentiated us, and the optimism he expressed is of a general nature available to all and applicable to all things. That he invoked such optimism does not disclose whether he genuinely believes that AIDS can be stopped if only we all come together. He did, however, vow to continue funding research at unprecedented levels. For all his general beliefs in a limited role of government, George Bush obviously put more hope for the control of the epidemic in federally supported institutions in the rolling Maryland hills of Bethesda than in the political and cultural efforts of individual AIDS activists.

The Independent Candidate

Ross Perot's campaign for president was unorthodox in many ways. That he at one point withdrew from the campaign was typical of his unorthodox style. That he reentered the race just in time to participate in the October debate lent his presence there an energy unavailable to the other candidates. Perot's remarks about AIDS were brief, but they bear consideration. Given the initial question put to President Bush, Perot might have commented on the display of the Names Project Memorial Quilt taking place in Washington, D.C., at about that time, but he did not. Neither did he comment on Earvin Johnson's leaving the national AIDS commission. Instead, he began by paying the president a compliment:

> First, I think Mary Fisher was a great choice; we're lucky to have her heading the commission. Secondly, I think one thing—if we're set to do the job, I would sit down with FDA, look exactly where we are. Then I would really focus on let's get these things out.
>
> If you're going to die, you don't have to go through this ten-year cycle the FDA goes through on new drugs. I believe the people with AIDS are more than willing to take that risk, and we could be moving out to the human population a whole lot faster than we are on some of these new drugs. So I would think we could expedite the problem there.

Perot made an error of fact when he said that Mary Fisher was appointed by Bush to head the national AIDS commission. In fact, she was merely one member among others of that commission. Perot's compliment to Bush's wisdom in appointing her is impossible to read in a context where candidates are seeking voter advantage; it could be gratuitous or he may have offered that judgment merely as a segue from the president's remarks to his own. In either case Perot went on to discuss the AIDS epidemic primarily in terms of the drug approval process, giving the impression that the solution to the epidemic lies in greater speed in drug experimentation and evaluation. Given Perot's take-charge mentality, it is not surprising that he would want to sit down with the FDA to assess the state of drug development in the area. Not coincidentally, the question of expediting drug experimentation and approval for general use has been a central issue in AIDS activism from the beginning. Thus, in his solution to the AIDS epidemic—taming an unruly federal biomedical complex—Ross Perot also functioned as an accomplice of AIDS activists. Of course, neither Bush nor Perot would probably accept such a label, but in certain regards they shared similar goals. The brevity of Perot's remarks makes it difficult to ascertain what priority Perot thought should be given to AIDS research and treatment programs or whether the question of individual responsibility for avoiding HIV risk has any bearing on government responses to the epidemic. It is nonetheless clear that in many ways Perot thought AIDS no more and no less than another failing of contemporary government.

By contrast with Bush, Perot framed the problem of AIDS as soluble if only the efforts of the federal government were better coordinated, the bureaucracy controlled, and leadership of the president himself given over to a commitment to cure. This attitude forms part of Perot's general optimism that many, if not all of the problems facing the nation generally can be resolved by steadfast confrontation by persons brave enough to stare down bureaucrats and entrenched financial interests. Perot's AIDS optimism may therefore be less a commitment to the development of drugs than a function of his general antibureaucratic views. The problem of the HIV/AIDS epidemic in his eyes is really no different from other issues the government has simply failed to identify and address. Such an approach does not by itself implicitly or explicitly blame particular individuals for the epidemic. By contrast, the government remains the key player responsible for the health of Americans. Ineffective government is the key barrier to progress against the epidemic. This is a view that has had many soundings.

The Democratic Candidate

Bill Clinton began his remarks on AIDS in a conventional way, noting the number of PWAs and the number of dead thus far:

Over 150,000 Americans have died of AIDS, well over a million and a quarter of Americans are HIV-positive. We need to put one person in charge of the battle against AIDS, to cut across all the agencies that deal with it.

We need to accelerate the drug-approval process. We need to fully fund the act named for that wonderful boy Ryan White to make sure we're doing everything we can on research and treatment.

And the President should lead a national effort to change behavior, to keep our children alive in the schools. Responsible behavior to keep people alive. This is a matter of life and death.

I've worked in my state to reduce teen pregnancy and illness among children, and I know it's tough.

The reason Magic Johnson resigned from the AIDS commission is because the statement you heard from Mr. Bush is the longest and best statement he's made on it in public.

I'm proud about—I'm proud of what we did at the Democratic convention, putting two HIV-positive people on the platform, and I'm proud of the leadership that I'm going to bring to this country in dealing with the AIDS crisis.

Because the presentation was not a debate in a strict sense and because the question directed to George Bush asked him to offer an account of why people were dissatisfied with *his* leadership in regard to AIDS, Perot and Clinton were fairly free to offer what particular remarks they cared to make about the epidemic. Unlike Perot, Clinton did express dissatisfaction with Bush's leadership against the epidemic. Despite the formulaic compliment paid to Bush, Clinton suggested that Magic Johnson quit the national AIDS commission because Bush had ignored the epidemic—until the moment of this public forum.

Clinton did not, however, criticize any specific failures of the Bush administration. Instead, he offered four goals for his administration: (1) centralizing government efforts in one person, (2) speeding up the drug-approval process, (3) funding the measures introduced into Congress, and (4) leading with presidential visibility a national campaign to change behavior. The goal of centralizing leadership in one person has the attractiveness of all such efforts to coordinate the many and varied efforts of the federal government, to avoid duplication, and to maintain consistent priorities in all agencies. (Such efforts—recall the nation's energy and drug czars—have unfortunately not always had the kind of success desired.) Speeding the drug-approval process has a number of meanings all favorably viewed by AIDS activists: elimination of unnecessary bureaucratic delay, greater access to experimental drugs, and— most optimistically—symbolic if not actual advance toward an effective therapy if not an outright cure. Clinton also called for better funding of the congressional AIDS programs named in honor of Ryan White, the Indiana teenager who died with AIDS.

Clinton's fourth point bears detailed consideration. Reiterating Bush's concern about behavioral change, Clinton said that behavior should be changed and he suggested that an effective program against AIDS could not be conducted without the committed involvement of the nation's president. What specific kinds of involvement Clinton intended cannot be known from his short remarks, but by asserting the importance of presidential leadership in such a campaign he did imply that Bush and the president before him had failed to play such a role. Clinton also framed the issue as one of the protection of children, which is part of a conventional strategy of invoking the prosperity and health of future generations as incentives for current action. By asserting the importance of protecting children from AIDS, Clinton makes an entirely safe assertion: who, after all, could be against protecting children from AIDS? Such a future-oriented view, however, can justly be criticized for failing to appreciate the present toll of the epidemic. To the extent that the damages of the epidemic are construed as *future* damages, they remain underappreciated and may fail to galvanize the kind of efforts required to control the epidemic.

Clinton also recognized the difficulty of succeeding against the epidemic. He said, "I've worked in my state to reduce teen pregnancy and illness among children, and I know it's tough." Such an acknowledgment has a number of implications: that the program is likely to be costly, difficult to implement, and unable to fulfill all expectations. Acknowledging these limitations, of courses, raises the prospect of defeat but also realistically suggests a long and arduous but not impassable road ahead. Clinton certainly did not pose easy answers to the problem. Whereas Bush wanted to return the blame to individuals for putting themselves in the way of risk, Clinton's proposals all require concerted action with committed leadership and do not raise invidious distinctions between people with AIDS and people with other diseases. His proposals, however, could reconfigure "success" by limiting expectations.[8]

AIDS and Its Presidents

Ronald Reagan received blood transfusions after the 1981 assassination attempt on his life. Had that blood borne an HIV infection, the history of AIDS in the United States might have had a very different course. As it was, Reagan was not infected and his presidency can be judged as problematic in regard to leadership on AIDS. On the occasion of a 1985 AIDS benefit, for example, he sent a telegram expressing regret about Rock Hudson's diagnosis of AIDS.[9] In that telegram he also called on everyone to do what he or she could to stop AIDS. But the expression of regret and the challenge to care expressed in that telegram did not signal greater attention to the epidemic by Ronald Reagan. On the contrary, his call for everyone to do what he or she could to stop AIDS could even be understood as shifting the responsibility for the epidemic to gay men and drug users since Reagan did not offer the prestige of his office to lead the nation as a whole against the epidemic; he saw AIDS as something each person had to fight off. In large measure, Reagan's approach to AIDS was but a variant of his approach to drugs: "Just say no." Indeed, this approach often prevailed across the Reagan administration's responses to AIDS.[10] Against the backdrop of the presidential administration in which AIDS emerged, a presidential administration that saw AIDS as an individual struggle, subsequent presidential administrations could take many forms of coordinated social and government action and appear to be offering progress even if still moving forward slowly and in half-steps.

It has been widely acknowledged that the U.S. economy was the single most important issue in the minds of 1992 voters. AIDS might have figured prominently in economic analyses of the country during the presidential campaign, but it did not. In the first presidential debate George Bush did note how much money was going to AIDS research; Bill Clinton called for more funding, but he did not specify how much funding should be provided or how new funds might be available. No candidate otherwise addressed the costs of AIDS at that time. If the calculation that one and a quarter million people in the U.S. have HIV infection (to use Clinton's numbers) is correct, then approximately one out of every two hundred people here faces a life-threatening condition sooner or later. Such a figure makes no account of *new* cases of HIV infection which may be expected to occur since the time of those estimates. Such numbers certainly justify talk about how AIDS already is and will further be an economic crisis in its own right and how its challenges should be met. Some indication of how that economic crisis would be met by an extended Bush presidency came several days after the first presidential debate. At that time the Bush administration was ready "to urge the Supreme Court to rule that employers may cut health insurance coverage of workers who develop costly illnesses like AIDS."[11] Given that employer-based health insurance is the backbone of the health insurance system in the United States, such a move could "solve" part of the economic crisis of AIDS by limiting costs to employers. The effect would be merely to shift the costs to other quarters or abandon those persons with AIDS without alternative means of health coverage. AIDS is thus implicated in fundamental questions about the American economy, and it reveals in microcosm challenges to the equity of health-care financing in the United States. It is a telling judgment about the treatment of people with AIDS in the United States that the U.S. Supreme Court did in fact uphold a self-insured employer's right to limit health-care expenditures to persons with AIDS, limitations that require no advance notification.

If the purpose of the presidential debates was to detail the candidates' positions on vital issues, then the voting public did get glimpses of their differences on the subject of AIDS. George Bush professed himself confounded by the efforts of politicized extremists and was at a loss to explain how a prominent appointee to the national AIDS commission disappointed him. Yet he asserted that individuals (Mary Fisher) and institutions (the FDA) can utilize the rich financial resources the nation has marshaled in service of the fight against the epidemic. Ross Perot found in respect to AIDS the same kind of gridlock he found elsewhere in the federal government, implying that the solutions to the epidemic are possibly at hand but blocked by federal agencies unable to set aside partisan politics and standards of experimentation inappropriate for PWAs. He prefaced his remarks by saying "if we're set to do the job" in order to underline the importance of conscious resolve to address the problem, suggesting that the government has not yet steeled its resolve to act against AIDS. He faults government for failing to address the *seriousness* of the problem. Moreover, he noted the willingness of many PWAs to take bold chances, which has created the opportunity to bypass cautious and time-consuming methods of drug assessment. In contrast to the moderation that Bush counseled and the unclogging that Perot recommended as an antidote to everything Washingtonian, Clinton outlined a number of more specific recommendations that are in keeping with approaches often favored by Democrats. He included in those recommendations the need for forthright presidential involvement, though he also built into that call for urgent action a warning against excessive optimism about success.

The 1992 election gave Bill Clinton the opportunity and the challenge of translating his campaign pledges into government action. The evening of election day the president-elect addressed a crowd gathered in front of the old state capitol in Little Rock. In the second sentence of his remarks Clinton raised AIDS as a problem too long ignored.[12] He raised it at the head of a short list *even before* mention of the environment and defense spending. That kind of prominence for AIDS will be welcomed by many in the AIDS community. Many are optimistic at the onset of new presidential administration, and Clinton's rhetoric on the eve of his election was no doubt solace to those who found previous administrations wanting. Yet election eve rhetoric does not predict future action, and one may justly wonder whether such inclusiveness of AIDS into the mainstream of political rhetoric is not also a form of co-optation which might mask deficiencies in attention to the epidemic across the breadth of political culture. There are also questions of what place AIDS might have in the presidency of a man whose focus is on the economic revitalization of the nation, especially when that revitalization may call for considerable cuts in federal funding of research and treatment programs.

What If There Was an Epidemic and Nobody Came?

Not long after the inauguration of Bill Clinton in January 1993 the report *The Social Impact of AIDS in the United States* was released under the auspices of the National Research Council, part of the National Academy of Sciences. The authors of this report come from the humanities and social sciences disciplines (ethics, history, sociology, anthropology, theology) as well as from law, medicine, and economics. Their self-stated goal was "to capture and describe the process of impact and response of selected social institutions to the HIV/AIDS epidemic."[13]

Their findings, which have dealt a serious blow to AIDS activists working to stimulate public and governmental concern, may be summarized this way: unlike other epidemics which have "done great damage to social institutions," the HIV/AIDS epidemic "has not affected U.S. social institutions to any such extent." Despite the numbers of persons HIV/AIDS has affected, the report claims that the epidemic "had not significantly altered the structures or directions of the social institutions that we studied. Many of the responses have been ad hoc and may be reversed when pressures subside. Others may be more lasting, but only because they reinforced or accelerated changes already latent or budding within the institutions." The panel concludes that "the limited responsiveness of institutions can in part be explained because the absolute numbers of the epidemic, relative to the U.S. population, are not overwhelming, and because U.S. social institutions are strong, complex, and resilient," adding that "another major reason for this limited response is the concentration of the epidemic in socially marginalized groups."[14]

While the committee's goal was to assess actual impact—defined as "concentrated force producing change, a compelling effect"[15]—they do not shrink from forecasting the future of the epidemic. In fact, they suggest that the epidemic will more or less be "absorbed in the flow of American life" even as "its worst effects will continue to devastate the lives and cultures of certain communities."[16] They note again: "The convergence of evidence shows that the HIV/AIDS epidemic is settling into spatially and socially isolated groups and possibly becoming endemic within them."[17] The report points out that "AIDS has increasingly been an affliction of people who have little economic, political, and social power" and concludes that "HIV/AIDS will 'disappear' not because, like smallpox, it has been eliminated, but because those who continue to be affected by it are socially invisible, beyond the sight and attention of the majority population."[18] The panel's main conclusion is that "the HIV/AIDS epidemic has effected many transient changes in the institutions that we studied and relatively few changes that we expect to be permanent."[19]

Despite its gestures of charity, taken as a whole this report announces not the end of the HIV/AIDS epidemic but the end of the need for the majority (read: straight people and non–drug-users) to worry about it. The panel suggests that by and large American institutions have remained unchanged because not enough people have been affected by the epidemic and because those affected do not influence social institutions because they are socially marginalized from the outset. The treatment of rare and lethal conditions has proved difficult for health care professionals, but AIDS does not appear to have altered in any significant way the finance and delivery of health care in the United States.[20] Despite the extensive health care needed by some PWAs, the costs of AIDS have not proved unmanageable.[21] Problems that existed before AIDS—for example, the "dumping" of poor patients—remain problems now in the epidemic.[22] Drug-trial regulations have changed, even improved somewhat, but their ultimate goals and standards have not.[23] For all the discussion about the religious meanings of AIDS, most religious groups have not altered their bodies of belief. Given that the overall import of the report is to minimize the effect of the AIDS epidemic, it is not surprising that its publication was met with some expressions of apprehension. David E. Rogers, for example, who was vice-chair of the National Commission on AIDS, objected to the report this way: "I think there have been profound changes in American society." He lamented the "tragic" effect of the report,[24] which he feared would legitimize inattention to the epidemic, observing: "Many of us who have been working at the barricades on this disease have been trying to say that AIDS is a crisis. . . . Now this capable crew of people comes in with the blinders on and tells everyone not to worry anymore because it's only marginalized people who are affected."[25]

The principal question that may be posed about this report is whether the study question and methodology were in fact sensitive enough to pick up the enduring social impact of the epidemic—even if it is true that the main social institutions have "absorbed" AIDS. In one instance the authors fully concede that they may not have had access to what might be the most important information needed to draw conclusions about the significance of AIDS for religion: "the history of personal attitudes and actions of individuals who are informed and motivated by religious beliefs."[26] In other instances one seeks not missing evidence but rather missing questions. The report makes no attempt, for example, at a sustained measurement of changes in educational, media, and criminal and civil legal practices. Neither is there any focus on the epidemic's effect on the social institutions and culture of gay men and lesbians. The panel conducted no empirical studies on behavioral or attitudinal changes as a result of the epidemic.

While the National Research Council report describes and assesses AIDS as effecting few significant or enduring changes in the social institutions of this nation, it fails to provide any kind of benchmark by which such changes could or should be measured. The report does refer to bubonic plague and its influences, but that epidemic occurred in societies so historically and technologically removed from contemporary society as to be virtually irrelevant as a standard by which to measure the effects of AIDS in late twentieth-century society. The question then arises: if a communicable, lethal disease that affects approximately one out of every two hundred people is not capable of effecting durable social, institutional change, then what is? Or, to vary the question, what is the worth of documenting the ways in which AIDS does not effect that change?

In an essay of enduring worth, German philosopher Hans Jonas once pointed out that the kinds of ailments capable of mortally wounding a society are few indeed.[27] Direct challenges to the survival of a society itself are rare and must be devastating indeed. A well-organized society is by definition capable of absorbing a broad range of social assaults, morbidities, and mortalities. And AIDS has proved no exception as an example of disease a society can absorb. What made this National Research Council report possible was not changes in social institutions but the expectation of such changes, expectations fueled by a decade of inflammatory reports and their uncritical reception. Even if AIDS were much more communicable than it is, even if it were much more quick to kill than it is, still it might not fundamentally jeopardize social institutions or society itself. Even before the National Research Council report, we already knew this or should have known it. The question worth examining is not whether AIDS has jeopardized fundamental social institutions, but whether AIDS reveals ways in which those social institutions either contribute or perpetuate the epidemic by failing to provide the educational, medical, and legal supports whose absence weakens the resolve and capacity of men, women, and children to avoid HIV risks.

Panel members resisted interpretations of their report that suggested that AIDS was no longer worth worrying about. They responded on the contrary that the epidemic remains an important social problem, though one which will primarily affect limited populations. But unlike the Presidential Commission on the Human Immunodeficiency Virus Epidemic before it, this panel did not describe what kind of obligations a nation or specifically a government has for an epidemic of this kind. Certainly, the report does recognize the epidemic as an occasion and opportunity for reform,[28] but no priorities or specific recommendations follow from its conclusions. If the report is to be believed, the social obligation to work toward the end of the epidemic cannot be grounded in mortal threats to the existence of society, in morbid dangers to the public health of the society, or in any possible dangers to important social institutions. On the contrary, the obligation that emerges in response to the epidemic seems to be grounded in the obligation society has toward marginalized, disadvantaged groups. In other words, while there may be many steps a society wants to take in respect to HIV/AIDS efforts, its primary obligations in this regard derive from its duties toward the disadvantaged; the obligations thus belong to the domain of the supererogatory. The report functionally suggests that for the foreseeable future, the epidemic will so little change the theory and practice of social institutions in the United States that AIDS will have no special priority over all other troubles that afflict American society. Given the way in which other such "duties" have been ignored, and given the historical treatment of gay men and drug-users, it is not surprising that AIDS activists read this report as an "all clear" signal that society can return without worry to its preepidemic pleasures and preoccupations.

I wonder whether the panel's focus on the social impact of AIDS doesn't skew the problem of AIDS to the very same kind of "us" versus "them" mentality that prevailed through the first decade of the epidemic. The report has said, after all, "The convergence of evidence shows that the HIV/AIDS epidemic is settling into spatially and socially isolated groups and possibly becoming endemic within them."[29] This sentence could have been written exactly this way over a decade ago in reference to the *emergence* of the epidemic. By framing the question of the epidemic as a matter of its effect on social institutions the panel automatically excludes from consideration those persons whose lives cannot influence social institutions whether they are ill or healthy, whose lives are beyond the interest of social institutions. The report must of necessity then relapse into an "us" versus "them" dichotomy even as it tries to underline the importance of surpassing that distinction through charity.

The panel sometimes even reverts to the kind of homophobic language that so often prevailed in early discussions of the epidemic. For example, the report notes that AIDS "created a political environment that compelled the public health community to negotiate containment strategies with the population that was initially primarily infected—gay men."[30] This construction of events and its language of "compelled" and "political environment" suggest that the public health community should not have had to negotiate at all with anyone about "containment" strategies, except that gay men exercised undue influence in resisting such strategies. In this way the language positions gay men in general, not AIDS in particular, as the enemy of public health. Such a view reflects the way questions about control of the epidemic have also been questions about the control and social standing of gay men.

Political AIDS

If the National Research Council report undermines AIDS hysteria based on all-too-frequent forecasts of unimaginable social disaster, then certainly it will have achieved an important goal—though, oddly, not one identified by the authors themselves. Yet to the extent that this report sets the threshold of social disaster so high that only those catastrophes that fundamentally jeopardize the nature and function of social institutions count as disasters *obligating* society to react with all its resources and energies, it proves a disservice to the community of people affected by the HIV/AIDS epidemic. The attention this report gives to the increasing burden of HIV on the socially distressed is an important message, but that attention may be compromised by its moral and political implications about the obligations of society and government toward such persons. If AIDS does not command attention as a matter of survival or common good, the only justification for action against AIDS comes from voluntary efforts. Such duties could easily seem less pressing when considered against all the other obligations owed toward disadvantaged persons and society generally. In sum, the panel report leaves the moral duties of government unspecified. While professing to offer a disinterested social analysis, the report actually has the effect of structuring the future of the debate about attention to AIDS in education, funding, and national priorities. Not an AIDS manifesto, the report is nevertheless a political brief.

During the first 1992 presidential debate the candidates shared one particular view about the government's obligation in regard to AIDS. Each candidate acknowledged the central role of government for the development of effective anti-HIV therapies. The candidates' varying political philosophies and their understanding of the priority of AIDS in the national hierarchy did not alter that conclusion. Assuming that the candidates did not offer their views merely for tactical purposes, their conclusions on AIDS reveal a coalescence of their political and moral views, even an obliteration of the differences between their political and moral views on this topic. These kinds of political constructions regarding AIDS are instructive for the way they depict matters of human will and willfulness, the war between unseen viruses and human biology, and the obligations of government to citizens. It is worth remembering that the word *candidate* comes from the same Latin root as *candidiasis,* one of the defining conditions of an AIDS diagnosis. Romans running for election wore a distinctive *toga candida*—a white toga—in order to identify themselves to voters in an age before television and serious, dark-hued suits. Candidiasis is a white bacterial infection that affects the mouth, the esophagus, and even the brains of some PWAs. The observation that candidates and candidiasis share a common etymological origin should offer a reminder that AIDS cannot be constructed as an issue apart from the social and politicomoral forces in which it sickens, kills, and is used tactically in presidential campaign strategies and academic reports.

10

No Time for
an AIDS Backlash

Writing in *Time,* columnist Charles Krauthammer described the May 1990 protests by AIDS activists at the National Institutes of Health as a misdirected demonstration: "The idea that American government or American society has been inattentive or unresponsive to AIDS is quite simply absurd." On the contrary, he continued, "AIDS has become the most privileged disease in America" since Congress continues to allocate an enormous amount of money for research and for the treatment of people with HIV infections and disease.[1] Except for cancer, HIV disease now receives more research funding than any other illness in the United States, a priority Krauthammer maintains is out of proportion to its significance since AIDS kills fewer people each year than many other diseases. The "privilege" of PWAs Krauthammer also extends to access to certain experimental drugs, access unavailable to others.

Chicago Tribune columnist Mike Royko also challenged the view that there is government indifference to AIDS: "That might have been true at one time. But it no longer is. Vast sums are being spent on AIDS research. Far more per victim than on cancer, heart disease, and other diseases that kill far more people."[2] In his view the Gran Fury poster showing interracial and different- and same-sex couples kissing (see figure 4) had more to do with the "promotion" of homosexuality than with the prevention of disease. Views of this kind would not only put homoeroticism back in the closet, they would also assign AIDS a lesser standing in the social and medical priorities of the nation.

The sentiment that gay men with AIDS were being treated as a privileged class surfaced as early as 1983 even prior to the identification of its viral origins.[3] What is new now is the increasing prominence of this view in public discourse and its justifications. In *The Myth of Heterosexual AIDS* political writer Michael Fumento mounts a full-scale defense of the proposition that the AIDS epidemic has achieved national and medical priority all out of proportion to its dangers, especially since the disease will make few inroads against white, middle-class heterosexuals. Fumento writes in self-conscious sound bytes: "Other than fairly spectacular rare occurrences, such as shark attacks and maulings by wild animals, it is difficult to name any broad category of death that will take fewer lives than heterosexually transmitted AIDS."[4] Or: "Most heterosexuals will continue to have more to fear from bathtub drowning than from AIDS."[5] He also says that the mass mailing of the surgeon general's report on AIDS to every household "makes every bit as much sense as sending a booklet warning against the dangers of frostbite to every home in the nation, from Key West, Florida, to San Diego, California."[6] Because there is no looming heterosexual epidemic and because the nation has neglected other medical priorities by siphoning off talent and money for AIDS research, Fumento concludes that "the ratio of AIDS research and development spending to federal patient costs is vastly out of proportion to other deadly diseases." Fumento also believes that the priority assigned to AIDS will endanger the lives of other people: "The blunt fact is that people will die of these other diseases because of the overemphasis on AIDS. We will never know their names, and those names will never be sewn into a giant quilt. We will never know their exact numbers. But they will die nonetheless."[7]

Not only the priority of AIDS on the national agenda but also the tactics used to put it there and keep it there have found their critics. Krauthammer concedes that the gains made by AIDS activists are a tribute to their passion and commitment, but he believes that such gains have been won by deceptive strategies. He charges that the "homosexual community," to advance its own interests, first claimed that AIDS was everyone's problem because everyone was at risk and its solution required universal social urgency. As it became clear that people would not fall at random to the disease, he says activists changed their tactics and began to prey on social guilt: how dare a society let its gay men, needle-users, their partners, and their children sicken and die? But this guilt is unwarranted, Krauthammer believes, since for the most part HIV disease is the self-incurred consequence of ignoring clear warnings.

Also objecting to activist tactics, the *New York Times* criticized the ACT UP disruption that made it impossible for the secretary of health and human services to be heard during his remarks at the 1990 international AIDS conference in San Francisco.[8] "It is hard," the editors of that paper of record wrote, "to think of a surer way for people with AIDS to alienate their best supporters." They characterized the action as a pointless breakdown in sense and civility, adding that "ACT UP's members had no justification for turning a research conference into a political circus," especially since (in the standard refrain) society has not turned its back on people with AIDS but has committed extravagant effort and resources to the epidemic. The disruption, moreover, was deemed all out of proportion to the matters protested: immigration restrictions for people with HIV infection and President Bush's absence from the conference by reason of an event important to the reelection of North Carolina senator Jesse Helms.

In a different vein, English professor Bruce Fleming suggests in *The Nation* that Americans have come to hype AIDS because of a distorted sense of what it means to be sick and dying.[9] Westerners in general, he says, assume that the absence of disease is the normal state of human affairs; disease thereby becomes a divergence to be named, isolated, and eliminated. Thus there can be the fury and anger he found in a presentation at a Modern Language Association convention, an AIDS address full of discussions of Susan Sontag and Harvey Fierstein and laments about the lost golden age of free sex. Accepting sickness and death as an integral part of life, he thinks, would free us from the frenetic feeling that AIDS and all disease is unfair treatment amenable to moral and medical control—control that in any case is impossible to achieve.

Priority and Tactics

The criticisms mentioned above have some important messages—remembering people sick and dying with other conditions, keeping priorities and discourse rational, recalling the inevitable mortality of human beings as an antidote to their hubris—but I see little reason to shift the priority now devoted to the HIV epidemic, to smear the tactics that have made that priority possible, or to alter the view that sickness and dying with HIV disease are evils to be resisted.

Fumento makes the most direct claim that people are dying from neglect because the nation has chosen to worry about people with HIV. He argues that AIDS needs to be put into perspective, but he offers not a word about what priority an infectious, communicable lethal disease should receive as against, for example, diabetes or certain heart conditions, which are noninfectious and noncommunicable and can be successfully managed by medicine throughout life and which are also "preventable" by the kinds of behavior long known to extend health and life.[10] In fact, Fumento says nothing at all about how priorities ought to be set. Surely an infectious communicable, lethal disease affecting large numbers of people ought to receive priority over diseases that can currently be medically managed in a way that permits people to live into old age, a prospect not currently enjoyed by people with HIV disease. Whether funding should be allocated according to the number of persons affected by a particular disease is problematic, for such allocation would effectively orphan certain diseases altogether. Moreover, many of the diseases that do now kill people in numbers greater than AIDS have a *long* history of funding, and the expenditures made on behalf of AIDS research and treatment should be measured against that history, not solely against the individual lines of current annual budget allocations. In some ways, AIDS is only now catching up with comparable past expenditures.

Perhaps the seeming voluntary nature of infection invites the notion that enough has been done for those with HIV. Does the perception that HIV could be eliminated as a health worry if people simply avoided the sex and drug techniques implicated in infection drive public antipathy toward public expenditures for health care and research? It seems, according to this logic, that AIDS can be prevented even if not cured; by extension its costs should be equally preventable as well, especially since sex and drug use are under individual control. But HIV disease is not simply a matter of individual failure to heed clear warnings. Many cases of AIDS were contracted *before* any public identification of the syndrome itself. Even after the identification of the syndrome, there was no clear identification of its cause or how it might be avoided. Early in the epidemic there were no widespread efforts to protect blood used in transfusions, even when certain screening tests were available.[11] Even after the discovery of the presumptive viral cause and the development of blood-screening tests, educational efforts to reach persons most at risk were inadequate and in any case no one knew what forms of education were capable of effecting behavioral change. What educational programs there were have failed, then and now, to reach drug-users, their sexual partners, and persons in rural areas. Some persons were infected, of course, by means altogether beyond their control: by rape, by transfusion, by Factor VIII used in the control of hemophilia, through birth to an infected mother, by accidental needle infection from providing health care or using drugs, through artificial insemination, and so on. Because of ambiguities and delays (culpable or not) in biomedicine, education, and public policy, it is not evident for the majority of people with AIDS that there were "clear warnings" that went unheeded.

In any case, we must remember that the existence of such warnings now does not mean that they can be retrospectively applied to all persons in the past or that there will not continue to be people who fall outside the protection of educational umbrellas because of geography, chance, or accident. Over thirteen years have passed since the Centers for Disease Control first reported the occurrence of rare diseases in gay men and drug-using persons. Since that time another cohort of gay men and drug-users has come along, persons who may not have been educated about the dangers of HIV, young persons who will not yet have the maturity of judgment in sexual and drug matters, persons who may not have access to clean needles or drug rehabilitation programs, who may not have the personal and social skills necessary to avoid risk altogether. In some cases there may be cultural and social barriers to protection from risk as well, such as resistance to condom use, a reluctance grounded in the variable meanings of condom use.[12] We must remember too that in matters of sex and drugs, people are weak and not always capable of protecting themselves, even from the risks they know and fear. It is not surprising then that a considerable portion of *all* human illness is self-incurred, brought about through an individual's life choices. This is to vary the principle of the double-effect: what is chosen is not illness but sex, food, alcohol, drugs, and so on. The aftermath of these choices, unchosen if inevitable, may be illness. So considered, AIDS does not stand apart from, for example, the heart disease that is both the consequence of behavior amenable to choice and about which there is plentiful public warning. It would be idiosyncratic and therefore prejudicial to single out AIDS as undeserving of public attention and research unless one also made the equivalent claims about other diseases whose antecedents are in avoidable risk. A comparison of AIDS with other "avoidable" diseases might even show less sympathy for diseases like diet-related heart disease or smoking-related emphysema. These latter diseases can sometimes be seen as the result of thousands and thousands of badly made eating and smoking choices while an HIV infection can result from a single lapse in unprotected sex. To the extent that the avoidability of disease is thought relevant to judging its merit for social investment, it would seem in the example given that AIDS is less avoidable insofar as it involved only a single mistake whereas the other conditions had vastly more opportunities for avoidance and correction.

Where critics see misplaced privilege in the priority and attention AIDS has won they might instead see a paradigm for other successes. Should the priority accorded to AIDS research and care be seen as an indictment of the wiles of AIDS activists or should the rise of AIDS research and treatment be required study in schools of public health? AIDS activists are not trying to bleed the nation dry (though some would fundamentally redesign it), and neither are they blind to the nation's other needs. They are merely trying to ensure that government and medicine work together to achieve important goals. If other disease research is being neglected, the question is not whether activists have bullied the Congress or the American Medical Association into questionable priorities. The relevant question is why other health-care research services cannot be delivered with the urgency and high profile that the HIV epidemic has received. In this sense the HIV epidemic is an opportunity for critical thinking about the nature of health care in the United States: is it the nature of the disease itself or the design of the health-care system that makes the HIV epidemic so formidable? Is it the communicability of the disease itself or social attitudes toward sexuality and drug use that make prevention so difficult?

But all this talk of the priority given to the HIV epidemic can be misleading. AIDS is no privilege for anyone. A diagnosis of AIDS amounts to a virtually unlimited onslaught against an individual's physical, emotional, familial, and economic resources. In addition, there is the burden of stigmatization, given that the disease has been interpreted as a punishment or deserved consequence of immoral behavior. A 1988 report, for example, showed that, depending on the social category of the respondent, some 8 to 60 percent of persons surveyed considered AIDS to be God's punishment for immoral sexual behavior.[13] A minority of Americans is prepared to tolerate considerable discrimination against people with an HIV-related condition.[14] Varying but significant numbers of persons surveyed report that they would refuse to work alongside people with AIDS, would take their children out of school if a child with

AIDS were in attendance, would favor the right of landlords to evict people with AIDS, and so on. Perhaps the most telling results of a survey reveal that the majority of respondents believed health professionals should be warned if patients have an HIV infection; a third of these would allow physicians to decline treating such patients.[15]

This last observation would be benign by itself except that medical students and faculty are also expressing apprehension about working with people with AIDS and there is some evidence that some medical professionals are choosing specialties and geographies that will keep them at a distance from such patients.[16] Some physicians have even taken to the pages of the *New York Times* to announce that they will refuse to treat any patients with an HIV infection.[17] Nursing recruitment has become difficult for hospitals that care for large numbers of people with HIV. There are still places in the United States where hospital food trays are left at the doors of people with AIDS because the nutrition staff will not go into the rooms.

All the money thus far spent in the HIV epidemic has not by itself ensured adequate medical care for all people with HIV. This is especially true for the homeless who have HIV-related disease.[18] Neither have the dollars spent on HIV research produced any medical panacea. Improved treatment has proved important for many people but not for all, and there are still many unresolved questions about the long-term ability of key HIV therapies to extend the lives of all people with HIV infection or to guarantee a good quality of life.[19] Zidovudine notwithstanding, as Larry Kramer has pointed out, there continues to be one HIV-related death every twelve minutes in the United States.[20] Is it therefore surprising that ACT UP now chants, "One billion dollars . . . one drug . . . big deal"?

As sociologists Charles Perrow and Mauro F. Guillén point out in *The AIDS Disaster,* it is hard to "prove" that funding for AIDS research has been inadequate. But as they also point out a broad array of highly credible reports have each drawn attention to government and philanthropic failures to respond to the epidemic.[21] These reports have come from the Office of Technology Assessment, the Congressional Research Service, the General Accounting Office, the Institute of Medicine, the Presidential Commission on the Human Immunodeficiency Virus Epidemic, and the National Commission on AIDS. Whatever funding has occurred, it is hard to see that one can object to the amounts per se that yet need to be spent since the money called for, for example, by the presidential commission or the Institute of Medicine[22] is not an invented figure pulled out of the air as a way of keeping scientists and bureaucrats in fat salaries. The figures represent estimates made in good faith about the extent of funding needed. Early estimates calculated that billions would be required, and that estimation has not changed merely because headlines have moved on to other subjects. They should not change merely because the American public has decided that the money thus far spent has surpassed its interest in the diseases of gay men and drug-users.

Costs and Compensation

Perhaps some in American society question the amount of money spent on behalf of AIDS research and treatment because they are unfamiliar with the amounts of money that are already spent for biomedical research and treatment. The research carried out by the National Institutes of Health has always been enormously expensive, as has been the provision of medical benefits to veterans, the elderly, and the poor. The federal funding of dialysis for end-stage renal disease alone, for example, provides life-saving therapy for only some seventy thousand people yet its costs have been measured in the billions since Congress decided to pick up the bill for such services.[23] If this kind of funding is any precedent, neither high cost nor small number of affected persons serve as a convincing rationale for limiting the funding now accorded to AIDS research and treatment.

Budget requests based on what should be done are one thing, of course, and budgets actually produced in government legislative process are another. The question at issue in discussions about the "privilege" of AIDS is the question of what priority should be assigned to AIDS funding given all the other funding needs that face the nation. Richard D. Mohr has argued that AIDS funding exerts a moral claim insofar as the disease is associated with gay men, for in many of its most significant aspects the HIV epidemic among gay men is the consequence of prejudicial social attitudes and arrangements.[24] Because rituals, laws, educational systems, and prevailing opinion in the U.S. fail to offer gay men any clear or supportive pathway to self-esteem or any incentives to the rewards of durable relationships, society has effectively forced some gay men into promiscuous behavior. Neither does society permit gay men the opportunity to form families that could shoulder at least part of the care their sick need. Philosopher Patricia Illingworth has fleshed out this argument and extended it to drug-users as well.[25]

These are powerful arguments; it is hard to think of any public rituals in family life, education, the media, religion, or the law that dignify the love of one man for another or that support any abiding union there. Some cities now recognize domestic partner relations between gay men and between lesbians, as do some employers. But these arrangements are exceptions rather than the rule, and none of these existed during the early years of the epidemic. Promiscuity is sometimes used as the basis for an argument that gay men bring AIDS on themselves. But whose promiscuity is it anyway in a culture that does not offer public incentive or support to gay men for *anything but* socially invisible sexual relations? How can AIDS be blamed on gay men who pursue what social options are open to them? It is also hard to argue that society has protected its needle-users when it clearly cannot prevent drug use or offer successful drug rehabilitation programs. American society's enthusiasm for wars on drugs has not been effectively translated into action capable of helping any but a fortunate few stop their drug use. Needle-exchange programs have been rejected out of fear that such action will appear to condone drug use—a fear that is odd given the de facto acceptance of drug use by people at every level of American culture, including members of Congress, Supreme Court justice nominees, and presidents, as recent events have shown.

Isolated from the mainstream, and left to their own devices, many gay men, drug-users, their sexual partners, and their children find themselves at the mercy of an indifferent virus as they try to lead what lives they can. Diseases rarely "just happen." More often than not, society's economic structure and moral values permit them to happen, make them inevitable. Philosopher and bioethicist Robert M. Veatch has observed that fairness permits inequality of outcome where opportunities have been equal, but he has noted in health care "persons who are truly not equal in their opportunity because of their social or psychological conditions." Fairness does not apply "to those who are forced into their health-risky behavior because of social oppression or stress in the mode of production."[26] Because many of the persons who have contracted HIV have done so under prejudicial social arrangements, there is a significant argument that priority for HIV research and care is required as compensation.

But compensation alone does not constitute the sole moral imperative for society's obligation. Moral philosophy also avails itself of the supererogatory, those burdens we undertake beyond the call of formal obligation. The society worth praising, the society worth *having* is the one that finds ways to care and to research, even though there is no formal obligation to do so and for no other reason than empathy for its citizens who are ill and dying. The care of those who contracted HIV infection through blood transfusions or of women whose HIV was a result of a husband's sexual activity outside of marriage are examples of such responses. The morally admirable society would do what it could to protect such persons from infection and care for them when they are sick whether society specifically owed them this concern and care or not.

Because of its contributions to basic research in immunology and virology and because of its importance for the care of a great number of afflicted persons, AIDS research is as important as any other research being conducted in the United States today. Delaying this research will not only impede therapy and vaccine development but will also subject the eventual costs to inflation; AIDS research will only get more expensive the longer it is delayed. Delay also increases the number of people who will be potentially at risk of HIV infection. We should remember that in the history of the planet only one disease, smallpox, has ever been entirely eliminated;[27] every other disease known to humanity continues to take a toll. Bubonic plague, for example, is no stranger to the contemporary world.[28] HIV disease is a problem for our time and it will be a problem for future generations. It is not a disease at which one can throw a fixed sum of money before moving on. Even when fully effective vaccines and treatment become available, some people will fail to benefit from them by reason of social deprivation, geography, choice, or chance. HIV disease needs to be treated as a disease that is here to stay, not one that has already used its share of the limelight, the public coffers, and the public's indulgence.

Critics of AIDS activists's disruptions of traffic and speech seem to believe that quiet discourse argued in mannerly fashion by legislators consulting with medical boards is enough to ensure that the nation will set appropriate medical priorities. But this view of rationally framed public policy is not entirely true to history. There are few important social reforms that did not require the abandonment of polite discourse and the disruption of business as usual. Government and policy in this country have often been *as much* a product of protests, strikes, and civil disobedience as of reasoned debate. It is wrong to pretend that civil disobedience and social disruption are not part and parcel of this nation's political techniques, and it is wrong to blame AIDS activists for using them as others have. Perhaps we have forgotten that the United States owes its very origin to acts of rebellion that the *New York Times* might have found easy to condemn as breakdowns in sense and civility.

Without protests, moreover, one wonders how the battle against AIDS would have ever been launched.[29] In the early years of the epidemic the sickness and death of small numbers of gay men did not lend itself to the advocacy of important legislators and medical commissions. In some respects this state of affairs continues to this day. Most of the many recommendations of the 1988 *Presidential Commission Report on the Human Immunodeficiency Virus Epidemic,* for example, have done little but collect dust. If recommendations from a group with the stature of a presidential commission cannot spur action on important goals, what other recourse is there than the tried and true methods of protest which are as much a part of American democracy as its parliamentary rules of order?[30] It is a shame that critics see conspiracy, irrationality, and impropriety behind AIDS activism when they might see a standard of urgency and passion by which to evaluate and improve the entire health-care system in the United States.

In the context of broad health-care needs, the acceptance of dying that Bruce Fleming has urged seems an invitation to quietism. If disease and dying are inevitable, what incentive is there ever to resist? Granted, some Americans may have lost their sense of mortality, but I wonder what is to be gained in respect to biomedical priorities by restoring it. On the contrary, it may be the very perception of disease as "excrescence" that functions as the spur to its control and eradication. I see no point in glorifying disease and dying; the lessons they teach are easily learned and do not require advanced instruction. There is a point at which sickness and dying cease to offer insights into the human condition or opportunities for strength and become instead unbearable, unredeemable absurdity. To his credit Fleming does say that hesitation by the U.S. government to carry out necessary HIV research would be criminal. The change in the perception of death he counsels would thus hardly make any practical difference to the responsibility of government and medicine to resist the epidemic with all the resources it can muster.

The sentiment nevertheless grows that AIDS is getting more than its share of media attention, resources, and social indulgence. But there has been no diminution in the status of the epidemic to warrant a change in the scope or intensity of research and treatment programs. HIV remains a lethal, communicable virus. Despite better medical management, the number of HIV-related deaths continues to increase. More and more hospital resources have to be directed to the care of people with

HIV. What then accounts for the sentiment that AIDS is getting more than its share? From the onset of the epidemic there have been desperate prophecies about the toll of the epidemic and facile predictions that millions to billions would die.[31] Is it possible that critics say that AIDS has received more than its share because it has not yet killed *enough* people? Is the same indifference that first kept the epidemic at the margins of national attention now inspiring the claim that enough has been done? The sentiment against AIDS research and funding has been primarily argued in the popular press, not in professional journals of medicine, bioethics, or public policy. Can it be that this sentiment therefore belongs to those who do not know the epidemic at first hand, who are tired of gay men and drug-users in public view, who by their very distance from the epidemic can make the easy judgment that it is time to move on?

Setting Priorities

The question of how biomedical research and treatment priorities should be decided for HIV disease is extremely difficult. I offer the following discussion primarily to underline the need for sustained reflection on this problem but also to claim priority for HIV treatment and research, though that priority is neither unconditional nor exclusive.

It is truly difficult to demonstrate with any kind of fully convincing precision why certain biomedical research and treatment programs should have moral priority over others among the many worthy claimants for government dollars. The difficulty is compounded when the benefit of such research and treatment programs (for instance, for PWAs) is uncertain. Utilitarian counsels for promoting the greatest happiness for the greatest number of individuals prove an unreliable guide here because they are capable of subjugating the interests of some persons to a "greater" social good and because it is often unclear which among competing allocations will in fact promote the greatest happiness for the greatest number. For example, how might it be demonstrated that treatment and research for people with lung cancer would increase the greatest happiness of the greatest number in ways that treatment and research for people with AIDS did not? Moreover, certain diseases might be orphaned altogether under a utilitarian approach. Certain diseases, progeria, for example, strike only miniscule numbers of individuals. How could persons with progeria lay claim to any kind of biomedical priority according to this standard? Would not its claims be swamped by competition from the sheer numbers of persons suffering from other conditions, even less debilitating and less life-shortening conditions?

Meritocratic approaches to the treatment and research of diseases invite the invidious application of highly questionable standards about the worth of individuals. These approaches also suffer from the difficulties of establishing a morally convincing criterion of worth. How, for example, should a newborn with AIDS be judged as deserving or undeserving of treatment? After all, he or she has not yet "proved" any social worth. As another example, a man with AIDS may have served ably in the U.S. Congress. Might he not be said to deserve some support in recognition of that service, even if there were "immoralities" involved in his contracting an HIV infection? Meritocratic allocations of biomedical resources have proved offensive in the past, as in the case of renal dialysis,[32] and there is good reason to be suspicious of them as they are used in both the dispersal and denial of resources. The underlying question is whether meritocratic allocations advance a moral agenda at the expense of the vulnerable or at the expense of the diversity of "worthwhile" human life.

The meritocratic standard of allocation is especially problematic for PWAs. Many people hold PWAs responsible for their condition and judge them undeserving of social support. Strict libertarians too recognize no obligation on their part to "subsidize" the health care of PWAs; they might wish to contribute to charities to help treat and research HIV infection and disease, but they feel no obligation to do so. The former view ignores the way most persons are infected with HIV, that is, in ways that do not "deserve" the range of illness and disease that follow. Even if one grants for the sake of the argument that homosexuality and drug use are morally culpable, do they deserve either punishment as severe as AIDS or abandonment by the biomedical community? Is there any measure of proportionality in such a "punishment."[33] Moreover, biomedical research operates in ways that in a sense make these kinds of questions irrelevant. It would be a mistake to fail to research HIV pathogenesis merely because people sick with it "deserved" their infection and disease. Research, especially insofar as it may be expected to contribute to basic knowledge in immunology, virology, and neurology among other fields, does not gain by closing doors on research areas because the subjects are "unworthy." A libertarian willingness to contribute to biomedical support, as mentioned above, is wholly altruistic and not the enactment of a duty. While some individuals may be able to support their health-care needs insofar as biomedicine can treat their conditions, many people cannot. And most people certainly cannot afford to, by themselves or in conjunction with the donations of others, produce the biomedical research and experimentation necessary to discover treatments for conditions now untreatable. The health of a society in general and its biomedical progress can therefore prove ill-served by assuming that individuals only have obligations to themselves.

Because meritocratic approaches fail to be morally compelling guides, the allocation of resources for research and treatment could be governed by a presumption of equality in a population. Equality is an assumption necessary for the possibility of moral judgments themselves (otherwise people are merely forces antagonistic to one another), and equality is a powerful constitutional feature of U.S. political history. But a commitment to equality will not by itself solve scarcity problems. Indeed, depending on what one means by equality, such a commitment may aggravate research and treatment problems. If all persons with all diseases were treated as financial equals in terms of the health-care dollars available for treatment and research, individual health care would be seriously jeopardized and research programs crippled by a strictly egalitarian division of resources. But perhaps by equality we mean proportionality. The government would then expend its health-care dollars and research funds proportionate to the prevalence (or sometimes maybe even incidence) of a particular disability. Certainly there is an intuitive appeal to such a notion in that each group of people with a particular disease or disability knows in advance that allocation decisions are made proportionate to the gravity of the disease in the overall population. This kind of parity avoids the appearance that some diseases are treated preferentially while others are neglected. There is much to recommend this kind of approach, although again it cannot be and should not be expected to be the sole criterion by which allocation decisions are made. Such an approach would still need to consider, for example, the social significance of the disease or disability and take into account the likelihood of, for example, research success.

Philosopher Albert R. Jonsen has rightly noted that the traditions of medical ethics are often ill equipped to make decisions about larger social policies that affect distribution of health-care resources. The traditional emphases on patient protection, professional competence, and even altruism in the manner of the Good Samaritan cannot provide an unequivocal model for the rationing that is the irreducible consequence of finite human, material, and economic resources.[34] Seen in this light, the question of priorities for PWAs is not only a question that results from the emergence of a new disease syndrome but a question that becomes difficult because of the very limitations of the traditions of medical and social ethics, especially when these are strained by novel disease syndromes and the increasing costs of medical technology. We may then wonder whether questions challenging the priority given to HIV research and treatment aren't merely idiosyncratic, raised as they are about AIDS when they might also be raised about a whole range of other research and treatment priorities. And if they are idiosyncratic, might not their driving force be less disinterested analysis of social policy than homophobia, social disapproval of drug use, and contempt for the poor? Why, in other words, did questions about the general failings of social and medical ethics in establishing a convincing scheme of prioritization emerge with respect to HIV/AIDS when they might have equally well emerged with respect to resources allocated to, for example, veterans' health care unrelated to military injury or to subsidized renal dialysis?

As to the larger questions of how social policies ought to be arranged in respect of health-care resources, Jonsen observes: "Justice in health care has no actual patients: it seeks a principle of distribution that will, in anticipation of actual need, count some persons as worthy of attention and count others out."[35] And yet Jonsen is skeptical that such a principle can be identified. He rejects the notion of triage because the origin of that notion—returning soldiers to battlefield quickly—plays no role in contemporary thinking about the purposes of medicine.[36] He doubts, moreover, that any satisfying principle of rationing can be devised, not because—in the words of philosopher Alasdair MacIntyre—there is no neutral, independent standard of justice but because—in the words of ethicist Paul Ramsey—larger questions of social and medical priorities are "incorrigible to moral reasoning."[37]

There are many reasons to concur with the view that biomedical priorities are intractable to any simple moral ordering. For whatever values they might espouse, decision-making bodies such as legislatures and professional organizations are often driven by nonmoral considerations. Legislatures and professional groups are often large and lumbering institutions whose policies emerge for reasons as varied as the accidents of individual leadership, the force of social opinion, advice of legal counsel, administrative policies, economic considerations, or symbolic values. What is more important, the openness of human moral life to competing visions and standards does not even suggest the desirability of a single, unifying principle ordering all biomedical research and treatment in one lexical pattern. Biomedical research and treatment policies will always provoke uncertainty, an uncertainty that will sometimes frustrate those looking for help and funding but an uncertainty that will also preserve the flexibility of research and treatment and protect them from the rigidities of any single moral view about which sick people deserve help and which do not.

The use of moral philosophies to determine biomedical priorities in research and treatment is additionally problematic because such theories were not developed to address these kinds of questions. Even natural law traditions, which have always recognized the importance of maintaining health, do not easily lend themselves to questions of resource allocation. The question of biomedical priorities is complicated by nonmoral factors as well, especially when one takes research objectives into account. The progress of science cannot always be mapped or programmed in advance. Even well-plotted, well-financed research can fail to produce effective therapies. By contrast, important breakthroughs can take place in unforeseen, even accidental circumstances. There are therefore no guarantees that monetary priority will in fact lead to effective therapies or vaccines, let alone outright cures. The likelihood of success ought to be a factor in determining how money gets spent in both research and treatment, but it cannot be the sole criterion if one wants to leave the door open for those serendipitous events that play an important role in biomedical advance and if one acknowledges that even promising leads fail. The "spin-off" effects of research can also be expected to influence funding decisions since research can achieve many important secondary gains. Characterizing and ranking the relative importance of such possible gains in assigning moral priorities to competing research and therapy programs, however, poses questions of immense difficulty, especially when one starts to measure expected future benefits against the needs of living, suffering persons.

In spite of all these general difficulties in establishing priorities for biomedical research and treatment, I believe there are nevertheless several rationales for giving HIV/AIDS research and treatment high priority in funding. First, HIV is a communicable, lethal infection; it is not a self-limiting condition of only those now infected. It can be expected to appear in the children, sexual partners, and needle-sharers of those already infected for the foreseeable future. Second, given the wide prevalence and increasing incidence of HIV among persons who have claims to being socially mistreated, a claim of "compensatory damages" is certainly relevant in setting priorities.

John Rawls's contractarian account of justice as fairness is also relevant to the discussion here, especially his effort to identify the way in which society ought to be organized in favor of the most disadvantaged persons.[38] Rawls believes that conclusions about the social distribution of benefits can be drawn from a hypothetical circumstance he calls the original position. In the original position hypothetical persons are charged with identifying the broad principles governing social organization and access to resources and advantages. To ensure that their choices are fair he imposes on them a "veil of ignorance" that keeps them from knowing what role they would have in the society they are organizing. They must therefore try to secure advantages for all possible roles they might have once the veil of ignorance is lifted. Health and health care are important goods, but it is unclear in Rawls's account whether they are to be counted among the "primary goods" around which his governing principles are organized; they may nevertheless be profitably analyzed in the context of his general theory. On the one hand, people in the original position will recognize that they might be seriously ill or disabled when the veil of ignorance is lifted; they should thus wish to secure health-care entitlements from the society they are organizing. On the other hand, those same people will recognize that they might be persons who live in the full bloom of health and who have no significant need of health care; they will thus also want to protect themselves from having to pay for the health care of others. To use an example involving PWAs, people in the original position would understand that AIDS is a profoundly disabling condition often necessitating significant medical assistance. They would also understand that once the veil of ignorance is lifted, they might be gay men or drug-users at high risk of HIV infection or PWAs. From this perspective, a program of national health coverage for all medical needs might appear attractive. Yet these same persons would also recognize that they might be straight, non-drug-using individuals whose lives would not involve them in any significant HIV risk. Indeed, they might be blessed with a robust genetic endowment resistant to many kinds of disease. It would not be to the advantage of such a person to advocate the kind of costly nationally sponsored health care favored from the perspective of, say, poor drug-users with HIV infections. What kind of resolution is possible between positions so antithetical in what they would require of health care support? Because social disadvantages can be more damaging to people than social advantages can be rewarding, Rawls concludes that people in the original position would agree that the general construction of society ought to operate in a way that benefited the least advantaged. In this way, society could offset the disadvantages of, for example, poverty and ill health without unduly burdening others. It does not follow that all health-care needs would be met through favoring the most disadvantaged, but it does follow that the disadvantaged should have to be taken into consideration in the distribution of all society's resources.

It seems eminently reasonable to say that PWAs belong in the category of society's least advantaged persons. AIDS is a disabling array of disorders that puts one at significant risk of early death, and treatments are at the moment not only experimental in nature but are often beyond the economic and geographical reach of those who need them. While there has been advance in clearing away social hostility toward PWAs, still, as noted above, they often receive substandard treatment and social disapproval. It does not follow from this account that PWAs should be the first among those to benefit from a socially subsidized medical system. But it does follow that health-care resources ought to be apportioned in a way that devotes priority to those persons whose disorders most profoundly disadvantage them.

Another argument from the original position might recognize the duty to be charitable. This duty could make up the difference between what a society is morally obligated to provide by way of therapy and health care and the actual care and research people will in fact need. Thus persons who find themselves in full health outside the original position—indeed all members of society—would have some responsibility to meet the health needs of others as a matter of charity, whether through tax dollars, participation in biomedical research, organ donation, or other actions. This charitable duty would be an imperfect duty—it would belong to the individual person to exercise in accordance with his or her conscience, and no other person could demand the exercise of that duty. Nevertheless, a generalized, imperfect duty of charity which could be exercised in regard to the health care of others seems a reasonable outcome of the decision-making of Rawls's original position. The treatment of PWAs or biomedical research in regard to HIV would only have priority in fulfilling this duty to the extent that people with HIV were in fact among the most disadvantaged; charity exercised on their behalf would certainly meet any obligations imposed by a duty of charity. Since neither the provision of a minimal level of health care nor the recognition of a limited duty of charity would guarantee provision of all health-care treatment and research needs for PWAs, this position underscores too the importance of *individual* responsibility—to the extent possible—in pursuing therapy and promoting the kind of research necessary for one's individual disabilities. And this conclusion would extend to all forms of disability and disease.

The case for HIV/AIDS as a centerpiece for contemporary biomedical research and treatment allocations may be summarized in the following way. A Rawlsian moral consensus directs social and economic institutions to arrange themselves in order to benefit the least advantaged, and PWAs suffer the serious disadvantages of a communicable and lethal condition, putting them in that class of persons. A duty of charity may also be said to exist from a Rawlsian perspective, a duty that while not obligated exclusively to PWAs would certainly be met by efforts on their behalf. Notions that HIV/AIDS is a sanction for immoral behavior are unconvincing given that equivalent immoralities are not similarly punished. Even if HIV/AIDS were a divine punishment, there is no obvious justification for human contribution to that punishment or to its continuation.[39] There is also some sense in which AIDS treatment and research and treatment are owed to gay men, drug-users, and the poor as a kind of compensatory damage for social injustice or neglect contributing to the likelihood of their infection and lack of social protection, for example, the health insurance available to others. A whole range of other human disease is "self-incurred," so to view AIDS as undeserving of consideration on that account is merely and objectionably idiosyncratic. The arguments for such a priority for HIV/AIDS are not unconditional. Should advances in treatment diminish the illness of PWAs, their claim to priority in future research might be diminished against the competing claims of those with illnesses that have no equivalent therapy. Should the nation go to war, to use another example, biomedical funds might justly be withdrawn to finance that purpose. Should another novel, lethal syndrome appear or some nuclear disaster occur, such problems might also assume priority over the funding of HIV research and treatment. For these reasons it is better to see the arguments here not as establishing immutable duties to provide research and treatment for people with HIV/AIDS but as prima facie obligations. Perhaps it would be better still to see these arguments not as commitments required by the logic of moral duty but as counsels of supererogation.

The arrangement of biomedical priorities is and always will be guided by both moral values and pragmatic considerations. In addition, it will always be an awkward, ad hoc process. Nevertheless, there are reasons to maintain a priority for AIDS in research and treatment even if the often alarmist views about the eventual numbers of people expected to have AIDS prove unfounded. Perhaps one way to see the importance of HIV research is to consider what it would mean to diminish concern in this area. If HIV research and therapy are relegated to a lesser rank in the nation's priorities, it will be gay men, needle-users, their sexual partners, and their children who will continue to pay the price of neglect, and the epidemic may again become the shadow killer it was in the beginning. In view of the people who are still sick, who are dying, who bear the costs of this epidemic, it is too early and too shameful to say that enough has been done. It is certainly too early for a backlash.

Afterword

I belong to that generation that can remember two events vividly: first the announcement in 1963 that John F. Kennedy had been shot and, second, the news reports in 1981 about the unaccountable occurrence of rare diseases in gay men. I was in the fourth grade when the principal of my grammar school announced that President Kennedy had been shot. She then led the school in a decade of the rosary to pray for his recovery. Like many others, I vividly recall how the world at that time shrank in size to the black-and-white television images of Kennedy's funeral cortège proceeding to the national cemetery. Almost twenty years later I sat one summer night in Cambridge, Massachusetts, idly having a drink and reading a local gay newspaper. A brief one-paragraph article there summarized a report about rare diseases, *Pneumocystis carinii* pneumonia and Kaposi's sarcoma, in gay men in California and New York. I noted the item but didn't have much attention to give it; I was fully preoccupied with writing my dissertation and making plans to spend the fall in Europe. Even had I read the article more attentively, even had I read the original accounts in the *Morbidity and Mortality Weekly Report*,[1] I doubt I—or anyone—could have predicted how AIDS would change the world and future as much as or even more than an assassin's bullets.

Against a prevailing image of a future continually and increasingly despoiled of health and even public order by the epidemic, AIDS activists have contested biomedical and governmental policies they deem slow, punitive, and ineffective. In their protests they typically demand nothing less than an outright end to the epidemic. For example, AIDS activist Douglas Crimp has said: "We don't need to transcend the epidemic; we need to end it."[2] But there is reason to be cautious both about expecting that an end to the epidemic amounts to the end of all instances of HIV-related disease and that the goal of all AIDS activism is merely the end of the epidemic. An end to the epidemic, properly speaking, would not bring an end to all instances of HIV disease. In standard biomedical usage an epidemic is a pronounced or widespread increase of a disease against its normal background occurrence. A disease, therefore, is not epidemic because it causes a certain absolute number of deaths or because it decimates a stipulated percentage of an entire population. The term *epidemic* is reserved for specific upward variations in the normal or ordinary occurrence of a specific condition. A disorder need not take large numbers necessarily in order to count as an epidemic. Neither must a disorder kill in order to be considered an epidemic. An eye disease, for example, might be epidemic but kill no one.

Because the diseases that were grouped together as "AIDS" multiplied against an inconsequential prevalence, they have been an epidemic from the onset and will continue to be an epidemic as long as their numbers increase. AIDS will only cease to be an epidemic when its prevalence levels off over time, when the deaths from HIV-related causes equal approximately the number of new HIV infections. An end to the epidemic thus understood does not therefore mean that either infection or disease will altogether vanish. The end of the epidemic is compatible with the continued existence of HIV-related disease, new HIV infections, and death. The end of the epidemic and the end of HIV disease altogether are thus two separate matters. By drawing attention to the difference between the end of an epidemic and the end of HIV disease, I do not mean to open the door to quietism, to the belief that because disease is a part of the human condition, activists and biomedical researchers should abandon their struggles. On the contrary, I articulate this view about the permanence of HIV disease in order to caution against moral interpretation and social policy (and even some AIDS activism) that would view AIDS as a transient aberration in the health and politics of a culture, a view that indulges transient, "quick-fix" responses as adequate to meet the future of the epidemic. Unrealistic expectations about the end of the epidemic or the cure of AIDS may also prove unfortunate if the public and the politicians become disillusioned about such high ambitions and cease to confront the epidemic in the present. The future of the planet appears to be a future with AIDS, and all policy decisions about the epidemic ought to take into account the many ways in which the epidemic can prove intractable to short-term, ill-conceived, anti-AIDS measures that, for example, would try to curb the epidemic through punitive legal sanctions or educational measures that avoid mention of gay sexuality and drug use. The apparent permanence of AIDS also ought to disabuse some of the misconception that if only a select few individuals changed their wicked ways the future would be immunologically sound.

Another important lesson can be learned about the future of the epidemic not from looking at the statistical projections that are incessantly presented in discussions about the epidemic but from attending to the words of people with HIV themselves.[3] In June of 1991 Peter Adair's "Absolutely Positive" aired on PBS in Chicago. Greg Cassin, a man with HIV infection, said in that documentary: "I'm a human being. It's my right to have a shitty day. It's my right to have a cold. I'm a human being. It's my right to be a bitch. It's my right to be less than perfect. *It's my right to be HIV-positive.*"[4] In claiming the right to an HIV infection, Cassin wasn't claiming the right to be a public health immoralist. On the contrary, in the face of excoriations against "transmitting" the virus and "spreading infection" among the "innocent"; against relentless reminders about the lethal nature of HIV infection and the evils committed by PWAs; against exhortations to be unrelentingly strong in the battle against his infection; against the rally cries issued to end the epidemic; against interpretations making people with AIDS the linchpin for the evaluation of the worth, morality, and future of a nation, Cassin was merely asserting the right to be weak. It is a right that needs to be taken seriously as we think about the future of the epidemic, for human fallibility is just as central a fact of the epidemic as any biomedical description of the molecular properties of HIV.

The right to be weak generates the duty of others to respect the limits of human capacity. It is unfair to ask people to carry burdens they cannot bear; it is unfair to impose policies that cannot be carried out. Barring an unexpected breakthrough in research for a treatment or vaccine, HIV disease will be a permanent part of the catalog of human suffering. AIDS will certainly not be defeated by "get tough" measures whose attraction will diminish with passing years, rising costs, and the foreseeable inability of dramatic headlines to energize a public inured to the epidemic. It thus becomes important that the energy of anti-AIDS measures be sustainable, that it cross generations. Battles over the moral meanings of disease have been fought before. Such conflicts, as in the case of the moral meaning of syphilis,[5] were not so much won by one side or the other as eclipsed in significance as biomedicine rendered the condition controllable.[6]

Albert Camus's *The Plague* has been quoted often in regard to the reasons for resolve and determination in the face of the HIV/AIDS epidemic. Indeed, there is much to admire in that novel's Dr. Rieux's day-to-day fortitude and perseverance against the plague that fell on the city of Oran. But another aspect of that morally fertile text is germane to moral attitudes in the AIDS epidemic. As the city is freed of its plague, Dr. Rieux mounts a roof overlooking the sea and the town where the citizens are noisily celebrating: in a way the survivors were returning to their lives as if the plague had never happened. But Rieux does not condemn them for reverting in their new-born freedom to desires that knew no limits. Instead, in the city's raucous obliteration of the plague he discerns the strength, joy, and innocence of human life and he feels "himself at one with them" even as he recognizes that their—and his—joy is always imperiled, for the plague may come again.[7] Camus did not require that the fight against the plague become an everlasting siege against human desires for repose and self-indulgence. One of his characters even mocks the pride some people will take in having survived the plague and their trivialization of grief through memorials. As Camus's novel makes clear, the fight against the plague can breed vices and evils of its own, can undermine heroes as well as create them if there is no room for forgetfulness and freedom from having to play the hero.

"Absolutely Positive" is just one reminder to those of us who are old enough to remember that there was a time before this epidemic, a time in which no one could have predicted that it would fall to such persons as Greg Cassin to be the standard-bearer for all the many causes that get collapsed together in debate about AIDS. But, as he wisely observes, the "amazing angels" in this epidemic are the people who bear the illness and who care for the sick and dying here and now. And that tack may be the only way out of the epidemic: to help people in their individual struggles against sickness and infection. People have to be helped in the lives they live—as gay men, as drug-users, as wives of secretly sexually active husbands, as teenagers tempted mightily by sex and drugs—rather than "helped" in the procrustean lives some would impose on them as "solutions" to the epidemic. They must be helped to protect themselves whatever their sexual lives and drug habits. The AIDS epidemic has fallen, after all, on people without regard to their ability to cope with it.

People with HIV were not preselected for infection according to their capacity to be strong, articulate, and politically agile. On the contrary, this epidemic has fallen on people underequipped in these regards, people with lives already complicated by the trials of gay and bisexual identities, drug use, skin color, and gender.

Continuing the trend of eloquent last words established by Socrates at his death, many books about AIDS conclude by offering some elevated remarks about AIDS and the future of humanity. There are in fact many things yet to be said about the future of the human community and its accommodation of HIV, but in many ways the most important question to pose is not whether society will "conquer" or "interdict" AIDS, for, as I've said, there are reasons to be cautious that this can happen. On the contrary, the most important question is whether people will continue to resist base interpretations of the epidemic and at the same time find concrete ways to help people affected by and at risk of HIV. We must resist the epidemic without imposing moralizing solutions that are worse than the epidemic itself. And if we pursue control of the epidemic this way, perhaps there can come a memory-scarring event, just like the assassination of President Kennedy or the appearance of that 1981 *Morbidity and Mortality Weekly Report,* which people will remember as marking if not the end of AIDS itself then at least the end of AIDS moralizing, an event that will give people freedom to be fallible if not freedom from infection, freedom to be HIV-positive, freedom from atavistic moral conceits that AIDS is a mark of difference signaling death, ruin, and social decay.

Notes

Introduction

1. Such was the argument advanced in a meeting of the Joint Chiefs of Staff as they discussed President Bill Clinton's proposal to end the official ban on gay men and lesbians in the armed services. See Erich Schmitt, "Joint Chiefs Fighting Clinton Plan to Allow Homosexuals in Military," *New York Times,* 25 Jan. 1993, p. A1.

2. Alan Cantwell, *AIDS and the Doctors of Death: An Inquiry into the Origins of the AIDS Epidemic* (Los Angeles: Aries Rising Press, 1988), 18 and passim.

3. See Raanon Gillon, "A Startling 19,000-word Thesis on the Origin of AIDS: Should the JME Have Published It?" *Journal of Medical Ethics* 18 (1992): 3–4.

4. See U.S. Senate Committee on Labor and Human Resources, *AIDS Treatment Research and Approval* (Washington, D.C.: U.S. Government Printing Office, 1987). Also see James Harvey Young, "AIDS and Deceptive Therapies," *American Health Quackery: Collected Essays* (Princeton: Princeton University Press, 1992), 256–285.

5. Friedrich Nietzsche, "On Truth and Lie in an Extramoral Sense," in *The Portable Nietzsche,* ed. Walter Kaufmann (New York: Viking, 1968), 46–47.

6. Timothy F. Murphy, "Is AIDS a Just Punishment?" *Journal of Medical Ethics* 14 (1988): 154–160.

7. See Elisabeth Kübler-Ross and Mal Warshaw, *AIDS: The Ultimate Challenge* (New York: Macmillan, 1987), 24.

8. *Thinking AIDS* (Reading, Mass.: Addison-Wesley, 1988), 9–10. Another writer cast the benefits of AIDS in theological language. He called AIDS

a "cleansing," saying that not only is the emergence of AIDS understandable given contemporary mores but also that it "must needs come in order that redemption be wrought and righteousness be established." Kenneth L. Vaux, *Birth Ethics: Religious and Cultural Values in the Genesis of Life* (New York: Crossroad, 1989), 49. That same ethicist elsewhere argued that "AIDS victims suffer and die as an act of crucifixion for the sin of the world" ("The Moral Anguish of AIDS," *Chicago Tribune,* 18 Sept. 1987, sec. 1, p. 23).

9. Douglas Crimp, "AIDS: Cultural Analysis, Cultural Activism," in *AIDS: Cultural Analysis, Cultural Activism,* ed. Douglas Crimp (Cambridge: MIT Press, 1988), 3.

Chapter 1. The Once and Future Epidemic

1. Randy Shilts, *And the Band Played On: Politics, People, and the AIDS Epidemic* (New York: St. Martin's Press, 1987), 11.

2. Shilts's treatment of Gaetan Dugas has previously been discussed by Douglas Crimp ("How to Have Promiscuity in an Epidemic," in *AIDS: Cultural Analysis, Cultural Activism,* ed. Douglas Crimp [Cambridge: MIT Press, 1988], 237–271, esp. 241–246) and by Judith Williamson ("Every Virus Tells a Story," in *Taking Liberties: AIDS and Cultural Politics,* ed. Simon Watney [London: Serpent's Tail/ICA, 1989], 69–80).

3. See Alessandro Manzoni, *The Betrothed,* trans. Bruce Penman (Middlesex: Penguin Books, 1972), 597–598, 647, and Daniel Defoe, *A Journal of the Plague Year,* ed. Anthony Burgess and Christopher Bristow (Middlesex: Penguin Books, 1966), 167–168, 173–174.

4. See "How to Have Promiscuity in an Epidemic" (pp. 241–243) in which Crimp details some of the headlines on "Patient Zero" that followed the release of Shilts's book.

5. See, for example, Jacques Leibowitch, *A Strange Virus of Unknown Origin,* trans. Richard Howard (New York: Ballantine, 1985).

6. Ronald Bayer, *Private Acts, Social Consequences: AIDS and the Politics of Public Health* (New York: Free Press, 1989). Elsewhere Bayer has also speculated that possible future shifts in public and professional thinking might use AIDS as evidence in favor of a pathological interpretation of homoeroticism. See *Homosexuality and American Psychiatry,* 2d ed. (Princeton: Princeton University Press, 1987), appendix. Indeed, AIDS had already been used in that way. See James L. Fletcher, "Homosexuality: Kick and Kickback," *Southern Medical Journal* 77 (1984): 149–150.

7. Monroe Price, *Shattered Mirrors: Our Search for Identity and Community in the AIDS Era* (Cambridge: Harvard University Press, 1989), 108.

8. Price, *Shattered Mirrors,* 108.

9. Other dire predictions about the future of the epidemic have been listed in Michael Fumento, *The Myth of Heterosexual AIDS* (New York: Free Press, 1985), 301.

10. Shilts, *And the Band Played On,* 21–22.

11. Shilts, *And the Band Played On,* 196.

12. Shilts, *And the Band Played On,* 165.

13. James Miller, "AIDS in the Novel: Getting It Straight," in *Fluid Exchanges: Artists and Critics in the AIDS Crisis,* ed. James Miller (Toronto: University of Toronto Press, 1992), 258.

14. Shilts, *And the Band Played On,* 83, 136.

15. Crimp has observed how very differently Dugas might have been characterized. See Crimp, "How to Have Promiscuity in an Epidemic," 245 n. 8.

16. Shilts, *And the Band Played On,* 165; emphasis added.

17. Shilts, *And the Band Played On,* 246–247.

18. Shilts, *And the Band Played On,* 251.

19. See Mary Catherine Bateson and Richard Goldsby, *Thinking AIDS* (Reading, Mass.: Addison-Wesley, 1988), 44–45.

20. Shilts, *And the Band Played On,* 439.

21. Shilts, *And the Band Played On,* 439.

22. Shilts, *And the Band Played On,* 147.

23. Shilts, *And the Band Played On,* 147.

24. Shilts, *And the Band Played On,* 147.

25. For an analysis of the way the "fast lane" may be an artifact of social oppression of gay men, see Patricia Illingworth, *AIDS and the Good Society* (London: Routledge, 1990).

26. Price, *Shattered Mirrors,* 102.

27. Bayer, *Private Acts,* 4–5.

28. Bayer, *Private Acts,* 153.

29. Bayer, *Private Acts,* 241.

30. It is worth pointing out that it is not AIDS properly speaking (which is "merely" disease) but public opinion about the *meaning of AIDS* which will decide whether social and legal policies will change. By itself "AIDS"—understood as a constellation of pathogenic processes—is politically inert. The question is therefore not whether AIDS will change the future; the question is whether people will adopt interpretations of AIDS and its social significance that justify the kind of undesirable outcomes Price and Bayer are at pains to outline.

31. Richard D. Mohr, *Gays/Justice: A Study in Ethics, Society, and Law* (New York: Columbia University Press, 1988), 267.

32. Gene Antonio, *The AIDS Cover-Up? Real and Alarming Facts about AIDS* (San Francisco: Ignatius Press, 1986).

33. Antonio, *The AIDS Cover-Up?* 133.

34. Heta Häyry and Matti Häyry, "AIDS Now," *Bioethics* 1 (1987): 339–356.

35. Price, *Shattered Mirrors,* 96–97.

36. This conference was held in Amsterdam instead of Boston, as originally planned, in order to protest the United States ban on entry by persons with HIV infection. See chapter 5 for further discussion.

37. Lawrence K. Altman, "At AIDS Talks, Reality Weighs Down Hope," *New York Times,* 26 July 1992, p. A1.

38. "Selling Sex Does Not Pay," *U.S. News & World Report,* 27 July 1992, p. 52.

39. "Driving Blindly into an Epidemic," *U.S. News & World Report,* 27 July 1992, p. 54.

40. Lawrence K. Altman, "Cost of Treating AIDS Patients Is Soaring," *New York Times,* 23 July 1992, p. B8. See also both articles cited above (nn. 38, 39) in *U.S. News & World Report.*

41. "The Hidden Cost of AIDS," *U.S. News & World Report,* 27 July 1992, pp. 49–51.

42. Lawrence K. Altman, "AIDS-focused New Parties Are Proposed at Conference," *New York Times,* 20 July 1992, p. A2.

43. Lawrence K. Altman, "New Virus Said to Cause a Condition like AIDS," *New York Times,* 23 July 1992, p. B8.

44. Lawrence K. Altman, "'AIDS' without Trace of H.I.V.: Talks in Amsterdam on Five Cases," *New York Times,* 22 July 1992, p. A1.

45. "AIDS Puzzle: No Cause for Panic," *New York Times,* 23 July 1992, p. A22. Some researchers immediately questioned the significance of this newly identified virus. See Lawrence K. Altman, "Two Experts Questioning Report about Possible New AIDS Virus," *New York Times,* 2 August 1992, p. A1.

46. Geoffrey Cowley, "Is a New AIDS Virus Emerging?" *Newsweek,* 27 July 1992, p. 41.

47. See Nigel Hawkes, "Britain under Threat from Most Virulent Strain of HIV," *The Times* [London], 23 July 1992, p. 2.

48. See, for example, Malcolm Gladwell, "Officials Respond Cautiously to Reports of Mysterious AIDS-like Disease," *Washington Post,* 22 July 1992, p. A4, and Cowley, "Is a New AIDS Virus Emerging?"

49. Peter Zingler, *Die Seuche: Roman* (Frankfurt am Main: Eichborn, 1989). For an extensive discussion of this work see Sander L. Gilman, "Plague in Germany: 1939/1989: Cultural Images of Race, Space, and Disease," in *Writing AIDS: Gay Literature, Language, and Analysis,* ed. Timothy F. Murphy and Suzanne Poirier (New York: Columbia University Press, 1993), 54–82.

50. See John Clum, "'And Once I Had It All': AIDS Narratives and Memories of an American Dream," in *Writing AIDS,* 219–221.

51. James Miller, "Dante on Fire Island," in *Writing AIDS,* 301.

52. Peter Bowen, for example, has faulted the film for its narrative movement to an increasingly insular, politically and socially isolated experience of AIDS rather than to an increasing confrontation of the racial, economic, and political circumstances of the epidemic ("Island Hopping," *OutWeek,* 16 May 1990, pp. 63–64).

53. Blaise Pascal, *Pensées,* trans. A. J. Krailsheimer (London: Penguin, 1966), 65.

Chapter 2. The Search for a Cure

1. Meurig Horton quotes Simon Watney to this effect in "Bugs, Drugs, and Placebo," in *Taking Liberties: AIDS and Cultural Politics,* ed. Erica Carter and Simon Watney (London: Serpent's Tail/ICA, 1989), 161.

2. Larry Kramer, *Reports from the Holocaust: The Making of an AIDS Activist* (New York: St. Martin's Press, 1989), 196.

3. See, for example, Lawrence K. Altman, "Government Panel on H.I.V. Finds the Prospect for Treatment Bleak," *New York Times,* 29 June 1993, p. B6; George Annas, "Faith (Healing), Hope, and Charity at the FDA: The Politics of AIDS Drug Trials," in *AIDS and the Health Care System,* ed. Lawrence O. Gostin (New Haven: Yale University Press, 1990), 183–194.

4. Paul Monette, *Borrowed Time: An AIDS Memoir* (New York: Harcourt Brace Jovanovich, 1988), 1.

5. Monette, *Borrowed Time,* 6–8.

6. Monette, *Borrowed Time,* 40.

7. Monette, *Borrowed Time,* 40.

8. Monette, *Borrowed Time,* 75.

9. I owe this comparison to Emily Apter's "Fantom Images: Hervé Guibert and the Writing of 'Sida' in France," in *Writing AIDS: Gay Literature, Language, and Analysis,* ed. Timothy F. Murphy and Suzanne Poirier (New York: Columbia University Press, 1993), 83–97.

10. Monette, *Borrowed Time,* 77.

11. Monette, *Borrowed Time,* 19.

12. Monette, *Borrowed Time,* 109.

13. Monette, *Borrowed Time,* 155.

14. Monette, *Borrowed Time,* 208.

15. Monette, *Borrowed Time,* 208–209.

16. Monette, *Borrowed Time,* 196.

17. Monette, *Borrowed Time,* 260–263.

18. On the history of sexual orientation therapy even after the APA decision to declassify homosexuality as necessarily a pathology, see Timothy F. Murphy, "Sexual Orientation Therapy: Techniques and Justifications," *Journal of Sex Research* 29 (1993): 501–523.

19. For example, see Joseph Nicolosi, *The Reparative Therapy of Male Homosexuality* (New York: Jason Aronson, 1992).

20. Monette, *Borrowed Time,* 3–4.

21. Bill Behrens, "AMA Bans Anti-Gay Bias," *Windy City Times,* 17 June 1993, p. 1.

22. Monette, *Borrowed Time,* 55.

23. Monette, *Borrowed Time,* 128.

24. Monette, *Borrowed Time,* 339–340.

25. Monette, *Borrowed Time,* 85.

26. Monette, *Borrowed Time,* 66.

27. "Founding Statement of People with AIDS/ARC (The Denver Principles)," in *AIDS: Cultural Analysis, Cultural Activism,* ed. Douglas Crimp (Cambridge: MIT Press, 1988), 148.

28. Monette, *Borrowed Time,* 335.

29. Monette, *Borrowed Time,* 103.

30. Paul Monette, *Afterlife* (New York: Crown, 1990).

31. David Wojnarowicz, "Living Close to the Knives," in David Wojnarowicz, *Close to the Knives: A Memoir of Disintegration* (New York: Vintage, 1991), 93.

32. Wojnarowicz, "Knives," 93–94.

33. Wojnarowicz, "Knives," 94.

34. Wojnarowicz, "Knives," 95–96.

35. Wojnarowicz, "Knives," 96.

36. Wojnarowicz, "Knives," 96.

37. Even prior to the emergence of AIDS, quackery had been a significant problem in U.S. health care. See James Harvey Young, *The Medical Messiahs: A Social History of Health Quackery in Twentieth-Century America* (Princeton: Princeton University Press, 1967). Reliance on sectarian medicine has also always drawn significant numbers of persons unhappy with orthodox allopathic medicine in the United States to osteopaths, chiropractors, folk healers, naprapaths, acupuncturists, and so on. See *Other Healers: Unorthodox Medicine in America*, ed. Norman Gevitz (Baltimore: Johns Hopkins University Press, 1988).

38. Wojnarowicz, "Knives," 107.

39. Wojnarowicz, "Knives," 107.

40. David Wojnarowicz, "X Rays," in Wojnarowicz, *Close to the Knives,* 114.

41. Wojnarowicz, "Knives," 115.

42. Wojnarowicz, "X Rays," 115–116.

43. Wojnarowicz, "X Rays," 118–119.

44. See Timothy F. Murphy, "Women and Drug Users: The Changing Faces of HIV Clinical Drug Trials," *Quality Review Bulletin* 17 (1992): 26–32.

45. Hervé Guibert, *To the Friend Who Did Not Save My Life* (New York: Atheneum, 1991). Guibert has also written *Le protocole compassionel* (Compassionate Access) (Paris: Gallimard, 1991), which continues the story of his quest for an AIDS cure.

46. Apter, "Fantom Images," 83.

47. James Miller, *The Passion of Michel Foucault* (New York: Simon and Schuster, 1993), 29.

48. Guibert, *To the Friend,* 13.

49. Guibert, *To the Friend,* 16–17.

50. Guibert, *To the Friend,* 23–24.

51. Guibert, *To the Friend,* 25.

52. Guibert, *To the Friend,* 31. See also James Miller, *The Passion of Michel Foucault,* 21.

53. Guibert, *To the Friend,* 39.

54. Miller, *The Passion of Michel Foucault,* 26–29.

55. Guibert, *To the Friend,* 222.

56. Guibert, *To the Friend,* 10.

57. Guibert, *To the Friend,* 32.

58. Guibert, *To the Friend,* 10.

59. Guibert, *To the Friend,* 34–35.

60. Guibert, *To the Friend,* 35.

61. Guibert, *To the Friend,* 38.

62. Guibert, *To the Friend,* 119–120.

63. Apter, "Fantom Images," 87.

64. Guibert, *To the Friend,* 142.

65. Guibert, *To the Friend,* 143.

66. Guibert, *To the Friend,* 160.
67. Guibert, *To the Friend,* 16.
68. Guibert, *To the Friend,* 210–211.
69. Guibert, *To the Friend,* 37.
70. Guibert, *To the Friend,* 70.
71. Guibert, *To the Friend,* 165.
72. Guibert, *To the Friend,* 188.
73. Guibert, *To the Friend,* 208.
74. Guibert, *To the Friend,* 246.
75. Guibert, *To the Friend,* 207. Monette (*Borrowed Time,* 328–329) had similarly encountered a physician with no time for hopeless cases of AIDS.
76. Kramer, *Reports from the Holocaust,* 222, 267–268, 275 (for example).
77. Kramer, *Reports from the Holocaust,* 277.
78. See a number of articles on this federal legislation in "Practising the PSDA," Special Supplement, *Hastings Center Report* 21 (1991): S1–S16.
79. See Jack Kevorkian, *Prescription: Medicide* (Buffalo, N.Y.: Prometheus, 1992), and Derek Humphry, *Final Exit: The Practicalities of Self-Deliverance and Assisted Suicide for the Dying* (Eugene, Ore.: Hemlock Society, 1991).
80. See the conclusions of a U.S. National Institutes of Health conference: Lawrence K. Altman, "Government Panel on H.I.V. Finds the Prospect for Treatment Bleak," *New York Times,* 29 June 1993, p. B6.
81. National Research Council, *The Social Impact of AIDS in the United States,* ed. Albert R. Jonsen and Jeff Stryker (Washington, D.C.: National Academy Press, 1993).
82. Shilts, *And the Band Played On,* 451.
83. Andrew Holleran, "New Complicities," *Christopher Street,* no. 165, 1991, pp. 6–8.

Chapter 3. Testimony

1. Richard Hall, "Gay Fiction Comes Home," *New York Times Book Review,* 19 June 1988, p. 1. For a leap into the sea, see Fritz Peters, *Finistère* (New York: New American Library, 1985 [originally pub. 1951]).
2. See David Leavitt, *Family Dancing* (New York: Knopf, 1984), *The Lost Language of Cranes* (New York: Knopf, 1986), and *Equal Affections* (New York: Weidenfeld and Nicolson, 1989); Robert Ferro, *The Family of Max Desir* (New York: Dutton, 1983); Armistead Maupin, *Babycakes* (New York: Harper and Row, 1984) and *Significant Others* (New York: Perennial, 1987); and Stephen McCauley, *Object of My Affection* (New York: Simon and Schuster, 1987).
3. Douglas Crimp, "How to Have Promiscuity in an Epidemic," in *AIDS: Cultural Activism, Cultural Analysis,* ed. Douglas Crimp (Cambridge: MIT Press, 1988), 240; emphasis in the original.
4. See Douglas Crimp "Mourning and Militancy," *October* 51 (1989): 3–18.

5. Arguing against the view of the Names Project quilt as a petition or as a collective story, Richard Mohr concludes that its panels have a sacralizing function in service of the individual. See "Text(ile): Reading the Names Project Quilt," in Richard D. Mohr, *Gay Ideas: Outing and Other Controversies* (Boston: Beacon Press, 1992), 105–128.

6. Barbara Peabody, *The Screaming Room* (San Diego: Oak Tree Publications, 1986).

7. Peabody, *The Screaming Room*, 248.

8. Andrew Holleran, *Dancer from the Dance* (New York: Morrow, 1978); see also his *Nights in Aruba* (New York: New American Library, 1983).

9. Andrew Holleran, "Circles," *Christopher Street*, no. 103, 1986, pp. 7–10.

10. Andrew Holleran, "Ernie's Funeral," *Christopher Street*, no. 108, 1988, pp. 7–11.

11. Andrew Holleran, *Ground Zero* (New York: Morrow, 1989), 201–209.

12. Holleran, *Ground Zero*, 91–99.

13. Holleran, *Ground Zero*, 73–80.

14. Holleran, *Ground Zero*, 29–36.

15. Andrew Holleran, "George Stambolian, Professor of Desire," *Christopher Street*, no. 173, 1992, pp. 3–5.

16. Holleran, *Ground Zero*, 29–36.

17. Peabody, *The Screaming Room*, 253.

18. Andrew Holleran, "Reading and Writing," *Christopher Street*, no. 115, 1987, pp. 5–7.

19. Paul Monette, *Borrowed Time* (New York: Harcourt Brace Jovanovich, 1988), 227.

20. *AIDS: The Women*, ed. Ines Rider and Patricia Ruppelt (San Francisco: Cleis, 1988), 31–35.

21. Elizabeth Cox, *Thanksgiving* (New York: Harper and Row, 1990).

22. Paul Monette, *Love Alone: Eighteen Elegies for Rog* (New York: St. Martin's Press, 1988).

23. Monette, *Borrowed Time*, 1.

24. Monette, *Borrowed Time*, 9–10.

25. Monette, *Borrowed Time*, 151.

26. Monette, *Borrowed Time*, 251.

27. Monette, *Borrowed Time*, 161.

28. Monette, *Borrowed Time*, 161.

29. Monette, *Borrowed Time*, 252.

30. "In Loving Memory of Jon B. Hettwer," *PWA Coalition Newsline*, no. 67, July 1991, p. 47.

31. Peabody, *The Screaming Room*, 7.

32. Monette, *Borrowed Time*, 88.

33. Cox, *Thanksgiving*, 76.

34. Cindy Ruskin, Matt Herron, and Deborah Zemke, *The Quilt: Stories from the Names Project* (New York: Pocket Books, 1988).

35. *Diseased Pariah News*, no. 3, 1992, p. 1. See "AIDS: Grin and Bear It," *Newsweek*, 15 Apr. 1991, p. 58.

36. Paul Rudnick's play *Jeffrey* is an example of the possibility of a comedy about AIDS. See Paul Rudnick, "Laughing at AIDS," *New York Times*, 23 Jan.

1993, p. A15, and Frank Rich, "Playwright Uses Laughter as Defense against AIDS," *New York Times,* 3 Feb. 1993, p. B1.

37. Holleran, *Ground Zero,* 11–18.

38. Gabriel Marcel, *The Philosophy of Existentialism* (Seacaucus, N.J.: Citadel Press, 1956), 91–103.

39. See Robert C. Solomon, *The Passions* (Notre Dame, Ind.: University of Notre Dame Press, 1976), 359–360.

40. Jeff Nunokawa, "'All the Sad Young Men': AIDS and the Work of Mourning," *Yale Journal of Criticism* 4 (1991): 1–13.

41. Nunokawa, "'All the Sad Young Men,'" 9.

42. After long refusal, the *New York Times* will now name lovers in obituaries. At the death of Enno Poersch, a cofounder of the Gay Men's Health Crisis, that newspaper reported, for example: "He is survived by his parents, Herbert and Ingeborg Poersch, and a brother, Ranier, all of Portland, Oregon. His companion was Michael Hatoff of Manhattan." See "Enno Poersch, 45, Dies; AIDS Group Founder," *New York Times,* 10 May 1990, B11.

43. Monette, *Borrowed Time,* 69, 83, 72.

44. Monette, *Borrowed Time,* 312.

Chapter 4. Celebrities and AIDS

1. George A. Gellert, Penny C. Weismuller, Kathleen V. Higgins, and Roberta M. Maxwell, "Disclosure of AIDS in Celebrities," *New England Journal of Medicine* 327 (1992): 1389. All citations are from this source.

2. Richard L. Madden, "McKinney Recalled as Fighter for the Poor," *New York Times,* 15 May 1987, pp. B1, B4.

3. Steven Lee Myers, "Anthony Perkins, Star of 'Psycho' and All Its Sequels, Is Dead at 60," *New York Times,* 14 Sept. 1992, p. D10.

4. Ryan White and Ann Marie Cunningham, *Ryan White: My Own Story* (New York: Dial Press, 1991).

5. Ronald Bayer, *Private Acts, Social Consequences: AIDS and the Politics of Public Health* (New York: Free Press, 1989), 191, 192, 196, 206.

6. Bruce Lambert, "Alison L. Gertz, Whose Infection Alerted Many to AIDS, Dies at 26," *New York Times,* 9 Aug. 1992, p. I50.

7. Philip J. Hilts, "Woman with AIDS Seizes Stage, Asking Bush to Help Ease Stigma," *New York Times,* 4 Aug. 1991, p. A1.

8. See Robert J. Blendon and Karen Donelan, "Discrimination against People with AIDS: The Public's Perspective," *New England Journal of Medicine* 319 (1988): 1022–1026, and Robert J. Blendon and Karen Donelan, "AIDS, the Public, and the 'NIMBY' Syndrome," in *Public and Professional Attitudes toward AIDS Patients,* ed. David E. Rogers and Eli Ginzberg (Boulder, Colo.: Westview Press, 1989), 19–30.

9. See M. Roy Schwartz, "Physicians' Attitudes toward AIDS" (pp. 31–41), Gayling Gee, "Nurse Attitudes and AIDS" (pp. 43–53), and Troyen A. Brennan, "Removing Barriers to Health Care for People with HIV-Related

Disease: A Matter of Law or Ethics?" (pp. 55–73), all in *Public and Professional Attitudes*. Also see Caryn Christensen, Ann King-Meltzer, and Barbara Fetzer, "Medical Students' Reaction to AIDS: The Influence of Patient Characteristics on Hypothetical Treatment Decisions," *Teaching and Learning in Medicine* 3 (1991): 138–142.

10. For a discussion of the ways in which such a presumption is already under siege, see Marc Seigler, "Confidentiality in Medicine: A Decrepit Concept," *New England Journal of Medicine* 32 (1982): 1518–1521.

11. H. Tristam Engelhardt, Jr., for example, describes the many conditions under which patients and physicians meet one another. It is worth noting that the fractured and transient nature of many health-care encounters in the United States suggests that neither patient nor physician should assume a commonality of views about the form and content of their relationship. Hence, a certain adversarial component may best protect the interests of both patients and physicians alike. See his *The Foundations of Bioethics* (New York: Oxford University Press, 1986), 256–262.

12. "Ashe has known he had AIDS since 1988, when doctors found an abscess on his brain caused by toxoplasmosis, an infection that is often a marker for AIDS. He and his wife, Jeanne, a fine photographer, decided not to go public with his illness for the sake of their daughter, Camera, who was two at the time. Ashe told a few close friends, who kept quiet. However, after *USA Today* informed Ashe this spring that it was pursuing the story, he felt that to maintain his privacy, he would have to lie about his health [if he denied the diagnosis]." Kenny Moore, "The Eternal Example," *Sports Illustrated,* 21 Dec. 1992, p. 26.

13. White and Cunningham, *Ryan White: My Own Story*.

14. Earvin "Magic" Johnson and William Novak, *My Life* (New York: Random House, 1992).

15. "Study Finds Many Heterosexuals Are Ignoring Serious Risk of AIDS," *New York Times,* 13 Nov. 1992, p. A10.

16. Nancy Collins, "Liz's AIDS Odyssey," *Vanity Fair,* Nov. 1992, pp. 208–213, 262–270.

17. The Arthur Ashe Foundation for the Defeat of AIDS, for example, raised $500,000 of its $5 million goal in only three months. Moore, "The Eternal Example," 21.

18. Kramer has written widely on the epidemic. Notable are his play *The Normal Heart* (New York: New American Library, 1985) and the autobiographical essays collected in *Reports from the Holocaust* (New York: St. Martin's Press, 1989).

19. James Miller, *The Passion of Michel Foucault* (New York: Simon and Schuster, 1993), 25. Foucault's death, as treated by Hervé Guibert, is treated by Emily Apter in "Fantom Images: Hervé Guibert and the Writing of 'Sida' in France," in *Writing AIDS: Gay Literature, Language, and Analysis*, ed. Timothy F. Murphy and Suzanne Poirier (New York: Columbia University Press, 1993), 83–97.

20. There was considerable litigation over the damages owed to Christian by reason of Hudson's failure to disclose. Christian was originally awarded virtually all of Hudson's estate (see "Hudson's Lover Wins $7 Million More," *New York Times,* 18 Feb. 1989, p. A7). The judge presiding in the case set that judgment

aside as excessive (see "Jury Award Is Sharply Cut in Hudson AIDS Suit," *New York Times,* 22 Apr. 1989, p. A7). Litigation continued even after these decisions.

21. Clifford D. May, "McKinney Dies of Illness Tied to AIDS," *New York Times,* 8 May 1987, pp. B1, B4. See also "AIDS Victim Rep. McKinney Dies," *Congressional Quarterly Weekly Report* 45 (1987): 899.

22. See Phillip Brian Harper, "Eloquence and Epitaph: Black Nationalism and the Homophobic Impulse in Responses to the Death of Max Robinson," in *Writing AIDS,* 117–139.

23. His cause of death was initially announced as bowel cancer. "Robert Reed, Actor, Dead at 59; The Father of 'The Brady Bunch,'" *New York Times,* 14 May 1992, p. B14.

24. "Journalist Randy Shilts Announces He Has AIDS," *Windy City Times,* 25 Feb. 1993.

25. See John Rockwell, "Rudolf Nureyev Eulogized and Buried in Paris," *New York Times,* 13 Jan. 1993, p. B8, and "A Lost Generation," *Newsweek,* 18 Jan. 1993, pp. 16–20, esp. p. 16. Nureyev's silence and his wish that his physician not disclose his diagnosis prompted gay writer Paul Monette to observe, "I don't consider him a great hero of the arts. I consider him a coward. I don't care how great a dancer he was" ("A Lost Generation," 19).

26. Bernard Weinraub, "Anthony Perkins's Wife Tells of Two Years of Secrecy," *New York Times,* 16 Sept. 1992, pp. C15, C17.

27. Weinraub, "Anthony Perkins's Wife," p. C15.

28. Glenn Collins, "Brad Davis, 41, A Leading Actor in 'Normal Heart' and 'Querrelle,'" *New York Times,* 10 Sept. 1992, p. B5.

29. Liberace's cause of death was originally reported by his physician to be congestive heart failure (see James L. Barron, "Liberace, Flamboyant Pianist, Is Dead," *New York Times,* 5 Feb. 1987, p. B6). After the county coroner ordered an autopsy, he declared that there was sufficient evidence to identify *Pneumocystis carinii* pneumonia as the cause of death (see "Omission of AIDS in Liberace Report Is Defended," *New York Times,* 14 Feb. 1987, p. A7).

30. Douglas Crimp, "Accommodating Magic," lecture presented at the conference, "AIDS: Images, Actions, Analysis," at the School of the Art Institute of Chicago, 1 Dec. 1992. Except for this paragraph, this chapter was written prior to Crimp's presentation.

31. "Travelers' Aids," *Hastings Center Report* 22 (1992): 2–3. Johnson's book is *What You Can Do to Avoid AIDS* (New York: Times Books, 1992).

32. See, for example, Arthur Ashe, "AIDS: Looking for Answers," *Proteus* 9 (1992): 1–2.

33. "Good Morning America," ABC, 1 Dec. 1992.

Chapter 5. The Angry Death of Kimberly Bergalis

1. For details of Rock Hudson's AIDS, see Randy Shilts, *And the Band Played On: People, Politics, and the AIDS Epidemic* (New York: St. Martin's Press,

1987), and Tom Clark and Dick Kleiner, *Rock Hudson, Friend of Mine* (New York: Pharos, 1989).

2. Johnson announced his diagnosis of HIV infection at a press conference in November 1991. See, for example, Erik Eckholm, "Facts of Life" and "The Long Road from HIV to AIDS," *New York Times,* 17 Nov. 1991, sec. 4, p. 1.

3. Centers for Disease Control, "Possible Transmission of Human Immunodeficiency Virus to a Patient during an Invasive Dental Procedure," *Morbidity and Mortality Weekly Report* 39 (1990): 489–493.

4. Hacib Aoun, "When a House Officer Gets AIDS," *New England Journal of Medicine* 321 (1989): 693–696.

5. Centers for Disease Control, "Update: Transmission of HIV Infection during an Invasive Dental Procedure—Florida," *Morbidity and Mortality Weekly Report* 40 (1991): 377–381. See more recently Carol Ciesielski, Donald Marianos, Chjin-Yih Ou, Robert Dumbaugh, Jon Witte, Ruth Berkelman, Barbara Gooch, Gerald Myers, Chi-Ching Luo, Gerald Schochetman, James Howell, Alan Lasch, Kenneth Bell, Nikki Economou, Bob Scott, Lawrence Furman, James Curran, and Harold Jaffe, "Transmission of Human Immunodeficiency Virus in a Dental Practice," *Annals of Internal Medicine* 116 (1992): 798–805. For a general discussion of the risk to patients from HIV-infected health-care workers, see Mary E. Chamberland and David M. Bell, "HIV Transmission from Health Care Worker to Patient: What Is the Risk?" *Annals of Internal Medicine* 116 (1992): 871–873.

6. Bruce Lambert, "Kimberly Bergalis Is Dead of AIDS at 23; Symbol of Debate over AIDS Tests," *New York Times,* 9 Dec. 1991, p. D9.

7. See Lambert, "Kimberly Bergalis."

8. See Lambert, "Kimberly Bergalis."

9. This view was evident in a personality magazine article that opined: "All who know her agree that Kimberly is the last person they would have thought might get AIDS." Bonnie Johnson, Meg Grant, and Don Sider, "A Life Stolen Early," *People,* 22 Oct. 1990, pp. 70–73.

10. In simple declarative form the headline asserts not that anybody can get AIDS but that no one is—can be—safe. This kind of inflammatory language is of a piece with alarmist pronouncements about AIDS which continue to this day.

11. Richard Mohr points out that the family in question here in fact belonged to a "high risk" group since the father was a hemophiliac, his wife had sex with him, and together they bore a child. See *Gays/Justice: A Study in Ethics, Society, and Law* (New York: Columbia University Press, 1988), 218–219. But indeed *all* the persons portrayed in the photoarticle were involved in "high risk" *behavior* since HIV infection is possible in all kinds of sexual intercourse, not merely same-sex intercourse. Moreover, even the "heterosexual" soldier featured in the article turned out to be lying to the magazine about not being gay. See Randy Shilts, *Conduct Unbecoming: Lesbians and Gays in the U.S. Military, Vietnam to the Persian Gulf* (New York: St. Martin's Press, 1993), 506–507.

12. "The New Victims," *Life,* July 1985, pp. 12–19.

13. "Gay Police Officer Infected with H.I.V. on Job, Judge Rules," *New York Times,* 8 June 1992, p. A16: "The ruling was hailed as a precedent that gay

public employees can overcome presumptions that AIDS always results from homosexual behavior."

14. See Sander L. Gilman, "AIDS and Syphilis: The Iconography of Disease," in *AIDS: Cultural Analysis, Cultural Activism,* ed. Douglas Crimp (Cambridge: MIT Press, 1988), 107.

15. See Gilman, "AIDS and Syphilis," 93–95.

16. Centers for Disease Control, "Recommendations for Preventing Transmission of Human Immunodeficiency Virus and Hepatitis B Virus to Patients during Exposure-prone Invasive Procedures," *Morbidity and Mortality Weekly Report* 40 (1991): 1–9.

17. See Johnson, Grant, and Sider, "A Life Stolen Early."

18. See Lambert, "Kimberly Bergalis."

19. See Robert J. Blendon and Karen Donelan, "Discrimination against People with AIDS: The People's Perspectives," *New England Journal of Medicine* 319 (1988): 1022–1026. See also "AIDS and the Real Electorate" [advertisement], *New York Times,* 24 Jan. 1988, p. A25.

20. This idea was suggested to me by Sander Gilman's "AIDS and Syphilis."

21. Mohr, *Gays/Justice,* 247–266.

22. See Johnson, Grant, and Sider, "A Life Stolen Early."

23. For an analysis of the meaning of *victim* see Jan Zita Grover, "AIDS: Keywords," in *AIDS: Cultural Analysis, Cultural Activism,* 17–30.

24. See Lambert, "Kimberly Bergalis": "When Ms. Bergalis's case was diagnosed, Dr. Acer told health investigators that he did not believe he had infected anyone."

25. This possibility was discussed, for example, on "Good Morning America," ABC, 11 June 1992, by George Bergalis, Kimberly's father, and another patient infected by David Acer.

26. See, for example, Max Navarre, "Fighting the Victim Label," in *AIDS: Cultural Analysis, Cultural Activism,* 143–145. See also James W. Jones, "Refusing the Name: The Absence of AIDS in Recent American Gay Male Fiction," in *Writing AIDS: Gay Literature, Language, and Analysis,* ed. Timothy F. Murphy and Suzanne Poirier (New York: Columbia University Press, 1993), 225–243.

27. See Lambert, "Kimberly Bergalis."

28. In her will Bergalis did leave $50,000 to the University of Miami Clinical AIDS research program and $10,000 to a local AIDS support group. See Paul Varnell, "AIDS Notes," *Windy City Times,* 23 Jan. 1992, p. 8.

29. "Good Morning America," ABC, 10 Dec. 1991.

30. See Navarre, "Fighting the Victim Label," 145.

31. Ann Landers, "The Positive Side of AIDS: A Fuller Life," *Daily News* (New York), 22 Dec. 1991, p. C20.

32. David Margolick, "For a Crusader Whose Time of Glory Has Come, Even AIDS Fails to Dampen the Spirit," *New York Times,* 5 Feb. 1993, p. B9. In the statement released after his death, actor Anthony Perkins said, "I have learned more about love, selflessness, and human understanding from the people I have met in this great adventure in the world of AIDS than I ever did in the cutthroat, competitive world in which I spent my life." See Bernard Weinraub,

"Anthony Perkins's Wife Tells of Two Years of Secrecy," *New York Times,* 16 Sept. 1992, p. C15.

33. For an argument against moralizing AIDS, see Eric Matthews, "AIDS and Sexual Morality," *Bioethics* 2 (1988): 118–128. See also Philip J. Hilts, "Dying Member of Panel on AIDS Wants Her Illness to Lift Stigma," *New York Times,* 4 Aug. 1991, p. 1, and Randy Shilts, "Good AIDS, Bad AIDS," *New York Times,* 10 Dec. 1991, p. A19.

34. If an HIV test were to be required of health-care workers, for example, should it be required after hiring or prior to hiring? And if it were carried out prior to hiring, would it be used to exclude job candidates from certain jobs?

35. Through the end of September 1993, a total of 339,250 cases of AIDS had been reported. See Centers for Disease Control, *HIV/AIDS Surveillance,* vol. 5, no. 3 (1993), p. 2.

Chapter 6. Health-Care Workers with HIV

1. American Medical Association, "AMA Statement on HIV-infected Physicians," 17 Jan. 1991.

2. In 1992 the board of trustees of the AMA withdrew this broad directive and in its place adopted an advisory that physicians should disclose an HIV infection to a state or local review committee which would then have the responsibility for making recommendations about any restrictions on the physician's practice. (American Medical Association House of Delegate Report, Report BB—"HIV Infections and Physicians," 1992.) This kind of reporting requirement is discussed below in chapter 7, "Teaching AIDS in China."

3. Centers for Disease Control, *HIV/AIDS Surveillance,* October 1993, table 3, p. 6, n. 5.

4. Jean Latz Griffin, "Edgar Signs Legislation on AIDS Notification," *Chicago Tribune,* 5 Oct. 1991, sec. 1, p. 1.

5. This was not the sole reason offered, however, since benefit of accurate patient diagnosis was also advanced as a reason for such testing.

6. Self-protection and protection of children are typically expressed concerns in this regard. See Mireya Navarro, "Patients Grilling Health Care Workers on AIDS," *New York Times,* 2 Aug. 1991, pp. B1, 2.

7. Navarro, "Patients Grilling Health Care Workers."

8. P. J. Burnham has parodied the possibility of full disclosure in his article "Medical Experimentation on Humans," *Science* 152 (1966): 448–450.

9. Centers for Disease Control, "Recommendations for Preventing Transmission of Human Immunodeficiency Virus and Hepatitis B Virus to Patients during Exposure-prone Invasive Procedures," *Morbidity and Mortality Weekly Report* 40 (1991): 1–9.

10. Centers for Disease Control, "Preliminary Analysis: HIV Serosurvey of Orthopedic Surgeons," *Morbidity and Mortality Weekly Report* 40 (1991): 309–312.

11. See chapter 5 above.

12. Rumors about doctors with AIDS often seem to have a life of their own, independent of facts. See, for example, "Coping with a Rumor That Could Be Ruinous," *New York Times*, 23 Jan. 1993, p. A7.

13. C. Mount and R. Kotulak, "Cook County Suspends Doctor with AIDS," *Chicago Tribune*, 3 Feb. 1987, sec. 1, p. 1. See too W. B. Crawford, "Doctor with AIDS Won't Be Restricted," *Chicago Tribune*, 25 Feb. 1987, sec. 2, p. 2.

14. H. Tristam Engelhardt, Jr., *Foundations of Bioethics* (New York: Oxford University Press, 1986), 250–335.

15. John Rawls, *A Theory of Justice* (Cambridge: Harvard University Press, 1971).

16. J. M. A. Lange, C. A. B. Boucher, C. E. Hollak, E. H. Wiltink, P. Reiss, E. A. van Royen, M. Roos, S. A. Danner, and J. Goudsmit, "Failure of Zidovudine Prophylaxis after Accidental Exposure to HIV-1," *New England Journal of Medicine* 322 (1990): 1375–1377.

17. It would remain an open question, of course, whether the information withheld would have altered a patient's choice. Nevertheless, such are the claims courts are asked to decide.

18. Such appears to be the conclusion of the court in a 1991 case. See David Orentlicher, "HIV-infected Surgeons: *Behringer v. Medical Center*," *Journal of the American Medical Association* 266 (1991): 1134–1137. See also an unpublished manuscript by Kenneth De Ville, "Nothing to Fear but Fear Itself: Informed Consent and HIV-infected Physicians," 1994.

19. Engelhardt, *Foundations of Bioethics*, 274.

20. Donald H. J. Hermann, "Torts: Private Lawsuits about AIDS," in *AIDS and the Law*, ed. Harlon L. Dalton, Scott Burris, and the Yale Law Project (New Haven: Yale University Press, 1987), 153–172.

21. Lawrence Gostin, "HIV-infected Physicians and the Practice of Seriously Invasive Procedures," *Hastings Center Report* 19 (1989): 32–39.

22. Norman Daniels, "Duty to Treat or Right to Refuse," *Hastings Center Report* 21 (1991): 36–46.

23. Monroe Price, *Shattered Mirrors: Our Search for Identity and Community in the AIDS Era* (Cambridge: Harvard University Press, 1989); Emily Apter, "Fantom Images: Hervé Guibert and the Writing of 'Sida' in France," in *Writing AIDS: Gay Literature, Language, and Analysis,* ed. Timothy F. Murphy and Suzanne Poirier (New York: Columbia University Press, 1993), 83–97; Ronald Bayer, *Private Acts, Social Consequences: AIDS and the Politics of Public Health* (New York: Free Press, 1989).

Chapter 7. Teaching AIDS in China

1. I adapt the phrase from Randy Shilts's characterization of Gaetan Dugas in *And the Band Played On: People, Politics, and the AIDS Epidemic* (New York: St. Martin's Press, 1987).

2. Jonathan Mann, "Worldwide Epidemiology of AIDS," in *The Global Impact of AIDS*, ed. Alan F. Fleming, Manuel Carballo, David W. FitzSimons, Michael R. Gailey, and Jonathan Mann (New York: Alan R. Liss, 1992), 6.

3. Shilts, *And the Band Played On*, 580.

4. "China Seen Alert and Active on World Aids Day," *China Daily*, 2 Dec. 1991, p. 3.

5. Max Navarre, "Fighting the Victim Label," in *AIDS: Cultural Analysis, Cultural Activism*, ed. Douglas Crimp (Cambridge: MIT Press, 1988), 143–146.

6. Sometimes, of course, the terminology is used not only to emphasize the plight of PWAs but also to underline the morally "innocent" status of, say, a baby, adolescent, or heterosexual adult with HIV.

7. There are suspicions that China has underreported the prevalence of HIV. See Philip Shenon, "After Years of Denial, Asia Faces Scourge of AIDS," *New York Times*, 8 Nov. 1992, p. A1: "Researchers say they believe that the number of Chinese infected with H.I.V. is much higher than the official figure released by the Government, which claims that only about 1,000 Chinese out of a population of 1.1 billion people carry the virus that causes AIDS. Because of intravenous drug use in China's southern provinces, H.I.V. infections are said to be growing at an explosive rate."

8. See Sander Gilman, "AIDS and Syphilis," in *AIDS: Cultural Analysis, Cultural Activism*, 87–107.

9. *Medical Journal of Australia*, vol. 1, no. 12 (1983): cover.

10. Charles M. Helmken, *AIDS: Images for Survival* (Washington: Shoshin Society, 1989), unpaginated.

11. Douglas Crimp and Adam Rolston, *AIDS Demo Graphics* (New York: Bay Press, 1990), and Douglas Crimp, ed., *AIDS: Cultural Analysis, Cultural Activism*.

12. See Richard Plant, *The Pink Triangle: The Nazi War against Homosexuals* (New York: Henry Holt, 1986).

13. See Crimp and Rolston, *AIDS Demo Graphics*. See, for example, Jeff Nunokawa, "'All the Sad Young Men,'" *Yale Journal of Criticism* 4 (1991): 1–13.

14. Billy Howard, *Epitaphs for the Living: Words and Images in the Time of AIDS* (Dallas: Southern Methodist University Press, 1989).

15. Peter M. Bowen, "AIDS 101," in *Writing AIDS: Gay Literature, Language, and Analysis*, ed. Timothy F. Murphy and Suzanne Poirier (New York: Columbia University Press, 1993), 140–160.

16. Gary Washburn and Robert Davis, "AIDS Poster Debuts, Fans Controversy," *Chicago Tribune*, 21 Aug. 1990, sec. 2, p. 3.

17. Robert Davis, "Three Call Special City Council Meeting on 'Kiss' Poster," *Chicago Tribune*, 21 Aug. 1990, sec. 2, p. 3. A *Chicago Tribune* editorial challenged the worth of the poster, saying that its message—purportedly that AIDS was not limited to gay men—got lost in "an AIDS campaign designed to create controversy over gay encounters. If it was an attempt to counter homophobia, certainly the brouhaha has had the opposite effect" ("Kissing Doesn't Tell Much about AIDS," *Chicago Tribune*, 17 Aug. 1990,

sec. 1, p. 22). Even some AIDS educators criticized the posters, though they did so anonymously, saying, "This poster does zip as far as AIDS education goes." One newspaper article even examined the claim that kissing doesn't kill and as evidence to the contrary reported the remote, theoretical, as yet unsubstantiated chance of HIV infection through kissing. See Jean Latz Griffin and Gary Washburn, "Experts Cast Doubt on AIDS Poster," *Chicago Tribune,* 17 Aug. 1990, sec. 1, p. 2.

18. This poster appears in Helmken, *AIDS: Images for Survival.*

19. Centers for Disease Control, "Recommendations for Preventing Transmission of Human Immunodeficiency Virus and Hepatitis B Virus to Patients during Exposure-prone Invasive Procedures," *Morbidity and Mortality Weekly Report* 40 (1991): 1–9.

20. For these reasons I voted with a small minority against this policy proposal.

21. Charles Perrow and Mauro F. Guillén, *The AIDS Disaster: The Failure of Organizations in New York and the Nation* (New Haven: Yale University Press, 1990).

22. Bret Hinsch, *Passions of the Cut Sleeve: The Male Homosexual Tradition in China* (Berkeley: University of California Press, 1991), 170–171. See also Fang Fu Ruan, *Sex in China* (New York: Plenum, 1991).

23. See Vincent E. Gil, "The Cut Sleeve Revisited: A Brief Ethnographic Interview with a Male Homosexual in Mainland China," *Journal of Sex Research* 29 (1992): 569–577.

24. "China Seen Alert and Active."

Chapter 8. HIV at the Borders

1. The impetus for such testing had been coming from a number of quarters during this time. See "Reagan Discloses Controversial AIDS Plan," *Congressional Quarterly Weekly Report* 45 (1987): 1210–1211.

2. See "AMA Opposes Reagan on AIDS Testing," *Congressional Quarterly Weekly Report* 45 (1987): 1381. While the AMA opposed mandatory testing in a number of instances, it did favor the testing of immigrants.

3. *Report of the Ellis Island Committee* (New York: Jerome S. Ozer, 1971 [originally pub. 1934]), 36.

4. Philip J. Hilts, "In Shift, Health Chief Lifts Ban on Visitors with the AIDS Virus," *New York Times,* 4 Jan. 1991, p. A1. In fact the headline here should have read "Health Chief Proposes Lifting Ban" because that proposal was never adopted.

5. Nancy Zeldis, "Senators Seek Change in Alien AIDS Policy," *National Law Journal,* 8 May 1989, p. 16.

6. Philip J. Hilts, "Clinton to Lift Ban on Visitors Carrying H.I.V.," *New York Times,* 9 Feb. 1993, p. A17; Clifford Krauss, "Immigration Ban on AIDS Is Backed," *New York Times,* 19 Feb. 1993, p. A7; Adam Clymer, "House, like

Senate, Votes to Ban Immigrants Carrying AIDS Virus," *New York Times,* 12 Mar. 1993, p. A8.

7. See Philip J. Hilts, "Landmark Accord Promises to Ease Immigration Curbs," *New York Times,* 26 Oct. 1990, p. A1.

8. Robert Pear, "Health Dept. Loses in AIDS Rule Dispute," *New York Times,* 28 May 1991, p. A18.

9. Karen De Witt, "U.S., in Switch, Plans to Keep Out People Infected with AIDS Virus," *New York Times,* 26 May 1991, p. A1.

10. De Witt, "U.S., in Switch."

11. Pear, "Health Dept. Loses."

12. Pear, "Health Dept. Loses."

13. Robert Pear, "Ban on Aliens with AIDS to Continue for Now," *New York Times,* 30 May 1991, p. A23.

14. "This AIDS Ban Invites Ridicule," *New York Times,* 19 June 1991, p. A24.

15. Harvey V. Fineberg, "False Aim against AIDS," *New York Times,* 31 July 1991, p. A19.

16. Lawrence K. Altman, "U.S. Ban of Infected Travelers Attacked at World AIDS Conference," *New York Times,* 17 June 1991, p. A13; Philip J. Hilts, "U.S. Policy on Infected Visitors to Keep AIDS Meeting Out of Country," *New York Times,* 17 Aug. 1991, p. A6.

17. Philip J. Hilts, "U.S. Policy on Infected Visitors." See Philip J. Hilts, "U.S. Planning to Allow Visits by People with AIDS," *New York Times,* 2 Aug. 1991, p. B2.

18. De Witt, "U.S., in Switch."

19. William Dannemeyer, *Shadow in the Land: Homosexuality in America* (San Francisco: Ignatius Press, 1989). Dannemeyer's title recalls former surgeon general Thomas Parran's book, *Shadow on the Land* (New York: Reynal & Hitchcock, 1937), which detailed for its time the social horrors of syphilis and, sometimes, the evils of syphilitics.

20. See Timothy F. Murphy, "Is AIDS a Just Punishment?" *Journal of Medical Ethics* 14 (1988): 154–160.

21. Pear, "Ban on Aliens with AIDS."

22. Margaret A. Somerville, "The Case against HIV Antibody Testing of Refugees and Immigrants," *Canadian Medical Association Journal* 141 (1989): 889–894.

23. I do not think the adoption of such a bar desirable; I make this point in order to underscore an inconsistency in attitude in the desire to protect U.S. citizens but not foreign nationals from possible HIV infection.

24. Indeed, there are many accounts that pinpoint the responsibility of Americans, specifically gay Americans, in exporting AIDS to other countries. For example, see P. D. Marsden, "AIDS: It Came for the Carnival," *British Medical Journal* 302 (1991): 337.

25. Clifford Krauss, "Immigration Ban on AIDS Is Backed," *New York Times,* 19 Feb. 1993, p. A7.

26. Margaret Somerville, "Law as an 'Art Form' Reflecting AIDS: A Challenge to the Province and Function of Law," in *Fluid Exchanges: Artists and*

Critics in the AIDS Crisis, ed. James Miller (Toronto: University of Toronto Press, 1992), 287–304.

27. Fineberg, "False Aim against AIDS."

28. "This AIDS Ban Invites Ridicule," *New York Times,* 19 June 1991, p. A24.

29. See David S. North, "Impact of Legal, Illegal, and Refugee Migrations on U.S. Social Service Programs," in *U.S. Immigration and Refugee Policy,* ed. Mary M. Kritz (Lexington, Mass.: Lexington Books, 1983), 269–285.

30. National Research Council, *The Social Impact of AIDS,* ed. Albert R. Jonsen and Jeff Stryker (Washington, D.C.: National Academy Press, 1993), 69.

31. See David F. Musto, "Quarantine and the Problem of AIDS," in *AIDS: The Burdens of History,* ed. Elizabeth Fee and Daniel M. Fox (Berkeley: University of California Press, 1988), 67–85.

32. Laurent DuBois, "Blood Stigma: Blaming Haitians for AIDS," *Proteus* 9 (1992): 20–24. See also Paul Farmer, *AIDS and Accusation: Haiti and the Geography of Blame* (Berkeley: University of California Press, 1992). On the connection with voodoo, see William R. Greenfield, "Night of the Living Dead II: Slow Virus Encephalopathies and AIDS: Do Necromantic Zombiists Transmit HTLV-III during Voodooistic Rituals?" *Journal of the American Medical Association* 256 (1986): 2199–2200.

33. Parran, *Shadow on the Land,* 36.

34. Philip J. Hilts, "U.S. Still Holds Haitians with H.I.V. in Cuba Base," *New York Times,* 10 Dec. 1992, p. A13.

35. See Michael S. Teitelbaum, "An Exodus Was Risky," *New York Times,* 2 Feb. 1993, p. A11.

36. Krauss, "Immigration Ban on AIDS Is Backed." As of this writing it is unclear whether the U.S. House of Representatives will affirm this vote or whether Mr. Clinton will veto any such measure put before him. As if to underline the homophobic implications of this kind of action, the media reported the Senate's action as linked to the president's efforts to lift the ban on gay men and lesbians serving openly in the military.

37. Mary B. Tabor, "Judge Orders the Release of Haitians," *New York Times,* 9 June 1993, p. B4. See also Thomas L. Friedman, "U.S. to Release 158 Haitian Detainees," *New York Times,* 10 June 1993, p. A6.

38. Somerville, "Law as an 'Art Form.'"

39. Musto, "Quarantine and the Problem of AIDS," 80.

40. For a review of some aspects of this exclusionary policy in force for about three-quarters of a century, see Peter N. Fowler and Leonard Graff, "Gay Aliens and Immigration: Resolving the Conflict between Hill and Longstaff," *University of Dayton Law Review* 10 (1985): 621–644.

41. See Anthony P. Maingot, "Ideology, Politics, and Citizenship in the American Debate on Immigration Policy: Beyond Consensus," in *U.S. Immigration and Refugee Policy,* 361–379.

42. This point was suggested to me by Judith Walzer Leavitt's, "'Typhoid Mary' Strikes Back: Bacteriological Theory and Practice in Early Twentieth-Century Public Health," *Isis* 83 (1992): 629.

43. Fineberg, "False Aim against AIDS."

44. Robert Pear, "U.S. to Argue Employers Can Cut Health Coverage," *New York Times,* 16 Oct. 1992, p. A14.

45. See "Health Insurance Horror," *New York Times,* 16 Nov. 1992, p. A12. The Supreme Court found an employer's action of setting a $5,000 lifetime limit on AIDS-related employee health benefits to be legal under the Employee Retirement and Income Security Act of 1974.

46. See Thomas J. Curran, *Xenophobia and Immigration, 1820–1930* (Boston: Twayne, 1975).

47. See Lawrence H. Fuchs, "Immigration, Pluralism, and Public Policy: The Challenge of the Pluribus to the Unum," in *U.S. Immigration and Refugee Policy,* 269–285.

48. Curran, *Xenophobia and Immigration,* 120–128.

49. Jean-Paul Sartre, *Anti-Semite and Jew* (New York: Schocken, 1948).

50. Michael C. LeMay, "U.S. Immigration Policy and Politics," in *The Gatekeepers: Comparative Immigration Policy,* ed. Michael C. LeMay (New York: Praeger, 1989), 1–21.

Chapter 9. Politics and Priorities

1. See "Where the Candidates Stand on AIDS," *Playboy,* Oct. 1987, pp. 50–51, 54, which compiles statements by Democratic and Republican presidential candidates in 1987.

2. That debate did not include all presidential candidates with views relevant to AIDS. Andre Marrou of the Libertarian Party, for example, opposed the ban on therapeutic marijuana use for the control of pain and nausea in PWAs. See Andre Marrou, "Why Gays Should Vote for a Libertarian President," *Windy City Times,* 15 Oct. 1992, p. 12.

3. "Transcript of the First Debate among the Presidential Candidates," *New York Times,* 12 Oct. 1992, pp. A12–15. All citations from this debate are from this source.

4. Fisher in fact represented the *third* heterosexual person to fill the position on the commission intended for someone with HIV. No gay man with AIDS was ever appointed to that post.

5. See James Harvey Young, *American Health Quackery: Collected Essays* (Princeton: Princeton University Press, 1992), 256–285.

6. See Jason DeParle, "111 Held in St. Patrick's AIDS Protest," *New York Times,* 11 Dec. 1989, p. B3. A PBS "P.O.V." presentation of the film that documented this protest, "Stop the Church," was canceled in 1991 because, according to a vice-president for scheduling and programming, the film "simply crosses the line of being responsible programming into being ridicule." The film's director, Robert Hilferty, denied that the film's intent was to ridicule; he said the "film followed the planning and outcome of the demonstration, in which 5,000 people gathered outside the church, and 134 of them entered and fell down in the aisles to symbolize death."

7. In fact, Bush once characterized the tactics used by AIDS activists as "an excess of free speech." See "Bush Assails Tactics Used by AIDS Lobby," *New York Times,* 21 Apr. 1991, p. I21. Bush had, of course, also cautioned against excesses by other protests. For example, while expressing sympathy for anti-abortion sentiments, he cautioned protesters in Wichita about excesses. See Maureen Dowd, "Bush Chides Protesters on 'Excesses,'" *New York Times,* 17 Aug. 1991, p. A7.

8. At both national Democratic and Republican conventions, speakers with HIV or AIDS addressed the audience. The 1992 Democratic party made AIDS visible in a way no presidential campaign had done before. Certainly, of course, the question of involvement of people with HIV at the convention raises the question of whether the speakers weren't co-opted from more direct and embarrassing confrontations with the political party. While such a perspective is possible because of the introduction of such persons into the campaign process, still the visibility—and especially the voice of people struck by HIV—countered the long lamented invisibility and voicelessness of PWAs in the national consciousness.

9. Nancy Collins, "Liz's AIDS Odyssey," *Vanity Fair,* Nov. 1992, p. 264.

10. Republican politician Jack Kemp, for example, observed: "But, as President Reagan pointed out, 'When it comes to preventing AIDS, don't medicine and morality teach the same thing?' All the research we have confirms that the answer to that question is 'Yes, they do.'" "Where the Candidates Stand on AIDS," 51.

11. "Health Insurance Cuts," *New York Times,* 16 Oct. 1992, p. A1; Robert Pear, "U.S. to Argue Employers Can Cut Health Coverage," *New York Times,* 16 Oct. 1992, p. A18. Ironically, the Court also held that the disabled may not be refused employment because of costs they would incur through insurance coverage. Robert Pear, "The Disabled Gain New Rights to Jobs and Health Insurance," *New York Times,* 9 June 1993, p. A1.

12. "Clinton: 'Tomorrow We Will Try to Give You Change,'" *Chicago Tribune,* 4 Nov. 1992, sec. 1, p. 22.

13. National Research Council, *The Social Impact of AIDS in the United States,* ed. Albert R. Jonsen and Jeff Stryker (Washington, D.C.: National Academy Press, 1993), p. 3.

14. *Social Impact,* 7.

15. *Social Impact,* 3.

16. *Social Impact,* 6.

17. *Social Impact,* 7.

18. *Social Impact,* 9, esp. 19.

19. *Social Impact,* 8.

20. *Social Impact,* 72 ff.

21. *Social Impact,* 74 n. 10.

22. *Social Impact,* 66.

23. *Social Impact,* 80 ff.

24. Liz McMillen, "Research Council's Report on AIDS Draws Fire for 'Insensitivity,'" *Chronicle of Higher Education,* 24 Feb. 1993, p. A9.

25. Chris Bull, "Report on AIDS Impact Draws Intense Criticism," *Advocate,* 9 Mar. 1993, p. 25.

26. *Social Impact,* 118.

27. Hans Jonas, "Philosophical Reflections on Experimenting with Human Subjects," *Philosophical Essays: From Current Creed to Technological Man* (Chicago: University of Chicago Press, 1993), 105–131.

28. For example: "The AIDS epidemic thus represents an opportunity and challenge for the revitalization of the practice of public health with regard to both infectious conditions and the chronic disorders that represent so much of the task of public health in the United States today . . ." *Social Impact,* 43.

29. *Social Impact,* 7.

30. *Social Impact,* 10.

Chapter 10. No Time for an AIDS Backlash

1. Charles Krauthammer, "AIDS: Getting More than Its Share," *Time,* 25 June 1990, p. 80.

2. Mike Royko, "Message on AIDS Gets Lost in Poster," *Chicago Tribune,* 21 Aug. 1990, sec. 1, p. 3.

3. See Randy Shilts, *And the Band Played On: Politics, People, and the AIDS Epidemic* (New York: St. Martin's Press, 1987), 295.

4. Michael Fumento, *The Myth of Heterosexual AIDS* (New York: Basic Books, 1990), 18.

5. Fumento, *Myth of Heterosexual AIDS,* 32.

6. Fumento, *Myth of Heterosexual AIDS,* 32.

7. Fumento, *Myth of Heterosexual AIDS,* 328.

8. "AIDS and Misdirected Rage," *New York Times,* 26 June 1990, p. A22.

9. Bruce Fleming, "A Different Way of Dying," *The Nation* 250 (1990): 446–450.

10. See Leon Kass, *Toward a More Natural Science: Biology and Human Affairs* (New York: Free Press, 1985), 157–186.

11. Shilts, *And the Band Played On,* 221, 308.

12. Dooley Worth, "Sexual Decision-making and AIDS: Why Condom Promotion among Vulnerable Women Is Likely to Fail," *Studies in Family Planning* 20 (1989): 297–307.

13. "AIDS and the Real Electorate" [advertisement], *New York Times,* 24 Jan. 1988, p. A25

14. Robert J. Blendon and Karen Donelan, "Discrimination against People with AIDS: The People's Perspectives," *New England Journal of Medicine* 319 (1988): 1022–1026.

15. Robert J. Blendon and Karen Donelan, "AIDS, the Public, and the 'NIMBY' Syndrome," in *Public and Professional Attitudes toward AIDS Patients,* ed. David E. Rogers and Eli Ginzberg (Boulder, Colo.: Westview Press, 1989), 19–30.

16. Theodore Feldman, Roger A. Bell, Judith J. Stephenson, and Frances E. Purifoy, "Attitudes of Medical School Faculty and Students toward Acquired Immunodeficiency Syndrome" (pp. 464–466); see also Charles J. Currey, Michael Johnson, and Barbara Ogden, "Willingness of Health Professions Students to Treat Patients with AIDS" (pp. 472–474); Thomas J. Ficarrotto, Margaret Grade, Nancy Bliwise, and Thomas Irish, "Predictors of Medical and Nursing Students' Levels of HIV-AIDS Knowledge and Their Resistance to Working with AIDS Patients" (pp. 470–471); all in *Academic Medicine* 65 (1990). On the choice of specialties, see Molly Cooke and Merle Sande, "The HIV Epidemic and Training in Internal Medicine," *New England Journal of Medicine* 321 (1990): 1334–1338.

17. Bruce Lambert, "AIDS War Shunned by Many Doctors," *New York Times*, 16 July 1990, p. A1.

18. Charles Perrow and Mauro F. Guillén, *The AIDS Disaster* (New Haven: Yale University Press, 1990), 166–169.

19. J. Ruedy, M. Schecter, and J. S. G. Montaner, "Zidovudine for Early Human Immunodeficiency Virus (HIV) Infection: Who, When, and How?" *Annals of Internal Medicine* 112 (1990): 1000–1002.

20. Larry Kramer, "A 'Manhattan Project' for AIDS," *New York Times*, 16 July 1990, p. A15.

21. Perrow and Guillén, *The AIDS Disaster*, 16 ff.

22. *The Presidential Commission Report on the Human Immunodeficiency Virus Epidemic* (Washington, D.C., 1988); Institute of Medicine, *Confronting AIDS: Update 1988* (Washington, D.C.: National Academy Press, 1988).

23. See John K. Iglehart, "Funding the End-stage Renal Disease Program," *New England Journal of Medicine* 306 (1982): 492–496. See also James E. Chapman, Ronald A. Sinicrope, and Douglas M. Clark, "Angio and Peritoneal Access for Endstage Renal Disease in the Community Hospital: A Cost Analysis," *American Surgeon* 52 (1986): 315–329.

24. See Richard D. Mohr, *Gays/Justice: A Study in Ethics, Society, and Law* (New York: Columbia University Press, 1988).

25. See Patricia Illingworth, *AIDS and the Good Society* (New York: Routledge, 1990).

26. Robert M. Veatch, "Voluntary Risks to Health: The Ethical Issues," *Journal of the American Medical Association* 243 (1980): 50–55.

27. Global Commission for the Certification of Smallpox Eradication, *The Global Eradication of Smallpox: Final Report of the Global Commission for the Certification of Smallpox Eradication* (Geneva: W.H.O., 1980).

28. C. T. Gregg, *Plague!* (New York: Scribners, 1978).

29. Herbert R. Spiers, "AIDS and Civil Disobedience," *Hastings Center Report* 19 (1989): 34–35.

30. Alvin Novick, "Civil Disobedience in Time of AIDS," *Hastings Center Report* 19 (1989): 35–36.

31. See Ronald Bayer, *Private Acts, Social Consequences: AIDS and the Politics of Public Health* (New York: Free Press, 1989), 3–4.

32. See Albert R. Jonsen, *The New Medicine and the Old Ethics* (Cambridge: Harvard University Press, 1990), 18, 46–47.

33. See Murphy, "Is AIDS a Just Punishment?"

34. Jonsen, *New Medicine and the Old Ethics*, passim.

35. Jonsen, *New Medicine and the Old Ethics*, 44.

36. Jonsen, *New Medicine and the Old Ethics*, 45 ff.

37. Jonsen, *New Medicine and the Old Ethics*, 48.

38. John Rawls, *A Theory of Justice* (Cambridge: Harvard University Press, 1971).

39. I owe this latter observation to Loretta M. Kopelman. See "The Punishment Concept of Disease," in *AIDS: Ethics and Public Policy*, ed. Christine Pierce and Donald VanDeVeer (Belmont, Calif.: Wadsworth), 49–55, and "Why Blaming the Sick Is Bad Medicine," *Medical Ethics for the Physician* 4 (1989): 5, 11.

Afterword

1. "*Pneumocystis* Pneumonia—Los Angeles," *Morbidity and Mortality Weekly Report* 30 (1981): 250–252, and "Kaposi's Sarcoma and *Pneumocystis* Pneumonia among Homosexual Men—New York City and California," *Morbidity and Mortality Weekly Report* 30 (1981): 305–308.

2. Douglas Crimp, "AIDS: Cultural Analysis/Cultural Activism," in *AIDS: Cultural Analysis, Cultural Activism,* ed. Douglas Crimp (Cambridge: MIT Press, 1988), 7.

3. For example, see Miriam Cameron, *Living with AIDS: Experience of Ethical Problems* (Newbury Park, Calif.: Sage, 1993).

4. Peter Adair, Janet Cole, and Veronica Selver, "Absolutely Positive" [film], 1991. Emphasis added.

5. See Suzanne Poirier, *Chicago's War on Syphilis, 1937–1940* (Urbana-Champaign: University of Illinois Press, forthcoming).

6. It is interesting to note that while biomedicine puts an end to certain moral disputes about meaning of disease, it also opens the opportunities for new ones. Medical control over syphilis diminished the way in which that disease was found suitable as an occasion for moral analysis, but biomedicine also demarcated new areas in which people might be found morally accountable for their illnesses. In identifying causal and merely statistical relationships between ill health and smoking, nutrition, alcohol use, exercise, and even medical examinations, biomedicine opens new possibilities in which people may be found culpable for "self-incurred" illness. Identification of the routes of HIV infection, for example, has been used to blame the infected for failing to protect themselves, as if mere cognitive knowledge about infection were a sufficient condition enabling protection from all risk across the variety of human lives.

7. Albert Camus, *The Plague* (New York: Vintage, 1972), 286–287.

Index

Absolutely Positive. See Peter Adair; Greg Cassin

Acer, David, 83; accused of intentionally infecting patients, 87; denies infecting patients, 88; identified as causing HIV infection in patients, 6, 200n5

Activism: as American tradition, 149; and anti-regulatory government, 148; criticism of, 148–149, 162, 163, 171–172; goals of, 49–50, 91–92, 167, 183–184; and obituaries, 62–66; poster art of, 113–117; protest at St. Patrick's Cathedral, 146, 148–149, 208n6

ACT UP, 28, 113, 115, 146, 164, 168. *See also* Activism

Adair, Peter, 185, 186, 212n4

Afterlife. See Paul Monette

AIDS: causes of, 17; communicability of, 23, 158, 167; control of, 15–19, 20; costs of, 135–138, 141–142, 168–169; culpability for, 14–15; cures for, 5; discrimination, 20, 71, 76, 167–168; education about, 76; effect of on social institutions, 156–157, 159–160; estimates of incidence and prevalence, 17, 21, 23, 94, 110, 151, 154, 202n35; funding for, 145, 149, 154; future of, 5, 11–12, 20*ff*, 152–153, 156–157, 184, 187, 191n30; as global terror, 21, 23; and homosexuality, 14–15, 17–18; idiopathic, 23–24, 192n44–48; meaning for ethics, 1–5; medical knowledge of, 16, 30–31; moral interpretations of, 185–186, 187; and nuclear holocaust, 21; origins of, 2–3, 5, 11, 12*ff*, 20, 111, 122, 159; punishment theory of, 3, 4, 167, 174; search for a cure of, 28*ff*, 39*ff* (*see also* Cure; Treatment; PWAs); and social obligations, 20–22, 40–41; stigmatization of, 31; theological views of, 3; underground, 36–38; vectors of, 14–15, 17. *See also* Cure; HIV infection; HIV testing

AIDS: Images for Survival. See Charles M. Helmken

The AIDS Cover-Up? See Gene Antonio

Al-721, experimental drug. *See* AZT

Albini, Cesar, 20

American Medical Association (AMA): advisory about disclosing diagnoses, 93, 202n1–2; policy on discrimination, 34; views on immigration policies, 205n2

American Psychiatric Association (APA), 33, 193n18

Amsterdam, 8th International AIDS Conference, 23, 132, 191n36

"Anointers," intending infection of others, 11
Antonio, Gene, speculation about AIDS, 21
Aoun, Hacib, 200n4
Apartheid in the cemetery, 65
Apter, Emily, 42, 45, 193n9, 194n46, 194n63, 198n19
"Arsenio Hall Show," 79
Ashe, Arthur: disclosure of AIDS, 76, 78, 82, 197n12; educational efforts, 77, 79, 81; fundraising efforts, 77, 79, 198n17
Asklepios, 24
AZT: experimental study of, 33, 39; uncertainties about worth, 45, 49

Bateson, Mary Catherine, 4, 191n19
Bathhouses, 15–16
Bayer, Ronald: images of the future, 12, 20, 190n6, 211n31; on rejection of "voluntarist" anti-AIDS measures, 20
Beijing Medical University, 108
Bergalis, George: denial of willful infection by dentist, 88, 201n25; view of daughter's infection, 86
Bergalis, Kimberly: infection of, 69, 82, 83; "innocence" of, 84, 87–88, 90–91; interest in HIV testing of health workers, 6, 82, 83; reaction to illness, 83, 87, 90; testimony before Congress, 83–84
Berlin, 9th International AIDS Conference, 49
Bill, American pharmaceutical executive, 45–47
Bisexuality, 88, 91
Blendon, Robert J., 197n8, 201n19, 210n14–15
Bob Damron's Address Book, 134
Borrowed Time. See Paul Monette
Boston, cancelled as conference site, 132
Bowen, Peter M., 192n52
Brennan, Troyen A., 197n9
Bridges, Fabian, 69
Buridan's ass, 46
Burnham, P. J., 202n8
Burris, Scott, 203n20
Bush, George: as AIDS activist, 7, 148; in campaign debate, 144, 145–149; criticism of activism, 146, 148–149,

154–155, 208n6, 209n7; on immigration policy, 130, 132; representation in AIDS poster, 116

Cady, Thomas, 85
Cameron, Miriam, 212n3
Camus, Albert, 186, 212n7
Canada, 136
Candidiasis, 161
Cantwell, Alan, 189n2
Carter, Erica, 192n1
Cassandra, 24
Cassin, Greg: "amazing angels," 186; right to be HIV-positive, 185
CDC. See Centers for Disease Control
Celebrities and AIDS: disclosure of diagnoses, 6, 69ff, 76ff; importance of involvement, 70, 76ff, 79; involvement in AIDS education, 70, 76; recruitment by physicians, 73–76, 80. See also Arthur Ashe; Kimberly Bergalis; Brad Davis; Perry Ellis; Michel Foucault; Paul Gann; Ali Gertz; Whoopi Goldberg; Rock Hudson; Larry Kramer; Liberace; Stuart McKinney; Rudolf Nureyev; Anthony Perkins; Robert Reed; Max Robinson; Randy Shilts; Elizabeth Taylor; Ryan White
Cemetery, 60
Centers for Disease Control (CDC): on emergence of AIDS, 33, 183, 187, 212n1; on exposure-prone procedures, 95, 119, 205n19
Chamberland, Mary E., 200n5
Chapman, James E., et al., 211n23
Chiang Kai-shek, 111
Chicago: controversy over Gran Fury poster in, 113–116; councilmen object to promotion of homosexuality, 113, 116, 204n17
China: attitudes toward HIV in, 110–112, 121–125; ethical problems in health care and, 109; incidence of AIDS in, 110–112, 204n7; merits of Great Wall, 110; poster art in, 117; student exercises in HIV policy, 7, 118–120; teaching experience in, 7, 108–109, 116–117; views on homoeroticism in, 122–123, 124; visitor policy regarding HIV, 109

Christensen, Caryn, et al., 198*n*10
Christian, Marc, 77, 198*n*20
Christopher Street, 54
Chwast, Seymour, 114
Ciesielski, Carol, et al., 200*n*5
Civilian War Dead in the United Kingdom, 64
Clark, Tom, 200*n*1
Clinton, Bill: in campaign debate, 146, 151–153; goals for his administration, 152–153, 155; policies of his administration, 139; pre-election views on HIV, 7, 130
Clum, John, 192*n*50
Coming out stories, 52
Confidentiality, 70
Congressional Research Service, 168
Cook, Molly, 211*n*16
Cope, Dennis, 35
Cosmo, had wicked sense of humor, 55
Cox, Elizabeth, 57, 58, 60
Crimp, Douglas, 8, 53, 79, 113, 184, 190*n*2, 190*n*4, 191*n*15
Cunningham, Anne Marie, 197*n*4
Cure: duty to seek, 49; existence of, 48, 50; meaning of search for, 32, 36–37, 40, 47, 48; obstacles to, 49, 194*n*37; social significance of, 20, 40–41, 48. *See also* Health care relations; Medicine; Placebo effect; Research methods; Treatment
Curran, Thomas J., 208*n*46
Currey, Charles J., et al., 211*n*16

Dalton, Harlon, 203*n*20
Dancer from the Dance. See Andrew Holleran
Daniels, Norman, 203*n*22
Dannemeyer, William E., 132–133, 134, 206*n*19
Davis, Brad, 78
Dear Abby, 23
Death, meaning of, 36, 51, 61–62, 66, 164, 172
Defoe, Daniel, 190*n*3
Dental care as cause of HIV infection. *See* David Acer
De Ville, Kenneth, 203*n*18
Disclosure of HIV/AIDS diagnosis: by celebrities, *see* Celebrities; by health workers, *see* Health care relations

Diseased Pariah News, 62
Donelan, Karen, 197*n*8, 201*n*19, 210*n*14–15
Drug users, 42, 53, 111, 112, 140, 166, 170
DuBois, Laurent, 207*n*32
Dugas, Gaetan: biography of, 12–13; characterized as Patient Zero, 11*ff*, 191*n*15; morality of, 13; moral judgment on, 13–14, 16, 19

Eddie, knew strip shows in New York City, 55
Education: acknowledging fallibility of, 151, 153, 165–167; homophobic aspects of, 18; obstacles to, 86; related to celebrity disclosure, 6
Elegiac art. *See* Testimony
Ellis, Perry, 77
Ellis Island, 129
Emigration: Jewish Soviets, 142; U.S. nationals with HIV abroad, 134, 206*n*23. *See also* Immigration
Engelhardt, H. Tristam, Jr., on health care relations, 101, 105, 197*n*11
Epidemic, defined, 184
Epitaphs for the Living. See Billy Howard
Equalitarian theory of resource provision. *See* Resource allocation
Ethics, nature of, 1, 3–5
Experimentation: access to experimental drugs, 148; expediting testing procedures, 148, 150, 157; record of achievement so far, 168; regulation of, 28, 148; relevance to disclosure of HIV infection, 100, 103
Explanation of evil, 27
Exposure-prone procedures, 95, 119, 205*n*19

Fallibility, meaning of, 185
Fang Fu Ruan, 205*n*22
Farmer, Paul, 207*n*32
Fee, Elizabeth, 207*n*31
Feldman, Theodore, et al., 211*n*16
Ferro, Robert, 195*n*2
Ficarrotto, Thomas J., et al., 211*n*16
Fierstein, Harvey, 164
Fineberg, Harvey V., 132, 141
Fisher, Mary, 145, 150, 155, 208*n*4
Fleming, Bruce, 164, 172

Fletcher, James L., 190*n*6
Food and Drug Administration (FDA), 148, 150. *See also* Experimentation
Foucault, Michel: death with AIDS, 69, 77; initial incredulity about AIDS, 43; knowledge of AIDS diagnosis, 44; views about death, 43
"Founding Statement of People with AIDS/ARC," 35
Fox, Daniel M., 207*n*31
Fuchs, Lawrence, 208*n*47
Fumento, Michael, 190*n*9; criticism of AIDS activists, AIDS education, and AIDS spending, 163; criticized, 165
Funerals, 54
The future: images of, 11–12, 19–27; significance of, 22, 24–26

Gang, poster work of, 116, 117
Gann, Paul, 69
"Gay cancer," 13
Gay men: affected by AIDS, 36–37, 54; associated with death, 64–65; exclusionary immigration policy, 140, 141; and identity, 14–15; leaping into the sea, 52; literature of and about, 52*ff*; obituaries of, 52*ff*; representations of, 14–15, 17; self-representations, 59–60, 65; social attention to, 163, 169, 170; vulnerability to AIDS, 15; without complaint, 15. *See also* Homophobia; Homosexuality
Gay-Related Infectious Disease (GRID), 13
Gee, Gayling, 197*n*9
Gellert, George A., et al., 197*n*1
General Accounting Office, 168
Gertz, Ali, 69
Gevitz, Norman, 194*n*37
Gil, Vincent E., 205*n*23
Gillon, Raanan, 189*n*3
Gilman, Sander, 192*n*49, 201*n*14–15, 201*n*20, 204*n*8
Global Commission for the Certification of Smallpox Eradication, 211*n*27
"God's country," 149
Goldberg, Whoopi, 77
Goldsby, Richard, 4, 191*n*19
Gostin, Lawrence, 203*n*21
Graff, Leonard, 207*n*40

Gran Fury, 113, 162, 204*n*17. *See also* Chicago
"Gray, Dorian," 39
Greenfield, William R., 207*n*17
Gregg, C. T., 211*n*28
GRID, 13
Gridlock, 155
Grover, Jan Zita, 201*n*23
Guantánamo, 138–139
Guibert, Hervé: nature of his writing, 42; representations of Foucault, 42; *To the Friend Who Did Not Save My Life*, 42–47, 194*n*45
Guide Michelin, 134
Guillén, Mauro F., 168, 211*n*21

Haitians: court rulings on, 139; in detention camp, 138–139; with HIV/AIDS, 138
Hall, Richard, 52
Harper, Phillip Brian, 199*n*22
Häyry, Heta, 21
Häyry, Matti, 21
HBV (hepatitis B virus), 120
Health and Human Services, Department of, 131, 133, 134
Health care institutions: affected by immigrants with HIV/AIDS, 7; burdens for public institutions, 136–137
Health care relations: adversarial components of, 100–101; AMA advisories about disclosure of diagnoses, 93; depersonalization in, 31*ff*, 43–44; diagnostic uncertainty in, 30–31, 39; HIV infection by dentist, 6, 69, 82; legislative oversight of, 83, 86, 88, 107; patient-physician relation, 30, 98, 100–101; physicians and the public health, 75–76; recruitment for causes in, 73–76; right to know about HIV/AIDS diagnoses in, 6–7, 93*ff*; testing for HIV, 6, 83, 86. *See also* Hacib Aoun; Health care workers; HIV testing; Homophobia
Health care workers: duty to treat PWAs, 168, 195*n*75; with HIV/AIDS, 94, 96, 108–109, 118–119, 202*n*10; infected occupationally, 94; obligation to disclose HIV/AIDS diagnosis, 6–7, 93, 94*ff*, 102, 103–107, 120–121; right to privacy, 97–98; testing

for HIV, 83, 118. *See also* China, student exercises on HIV policy; HIV testing

Heaven, perceived value of, 61

Heckler, Margaret, 49

Helmken, Charles M., 113, 204*n*10, 205*n*18

Helms, Jesse, 129, 130

Hepatitis B virus, 120

Hermann, Donald H. J., 203*n*20

Herron, Matt, 196*n*34

Heterosexual symbolism, 87

Hettwer, John B., 60

Hilferty, Robert, 208*n*6

Hinsch, Bret, 123, 205*n*22

HIV infection: immaculate, 89; moral meaning of, 86, 187; perception of communicability, 116, 124–125, 130, 131; right to, 185

HIV testing: anonymous, 70*ff*; and employability, 99, 118; and immigration policy, 129*ff*; limitations of, 1, 98; and the military, 2, 189*n*1; occupational infection, 85, 94, 200*n*13; and "panicked" testing, 71, 81; purposes of, 70, 87, 91, 202*n*5–6; as self-incurred, 147, 164, 165–166, 170, 174, 180, 212*n*6; testing policies, 3, 91, 94, 118–120, 202*n*34; use of test centers, 70–73. *See also* George Bush; Bill Clinton; Immigration

Holleran, Andrew: *Dancer from the Dance*, 54; *Nights in Aruba*, 54; testimonials, 54–56, 58; views on responsibilities for AIDS, 50–51; writing about AIDS, 62–63

Homelessness, 41

Homophobia: and blame for AIDS, 16–17, 79, 125, 160; in disclosure of infection and illness, 79, 95; in medicine, 29, 34–36

Homosexuality: alleged promotion of by AIDS poster, 113, 116, 162; in Chinese culture, 111, 122–123, 124; and immigration policies, 140; medical treatment of, 33; medicine's pathological views of, 33, 34. *See* AIDS, and homosexuality; Gay men; Lesbians

Hope, 27, 29, 36

Horton, Meurig, 192*n*1

Horwitz, Roger. *See* Paul Monette

Howard, Billy, 113, 204*n*14

Hudson, Rock, 69, 72, 73, 77, 82, 198*n*20

Hujar, Peter, 38

Humor and AIDS, 62

Humphry, Derek, 195*n*79

Iglehart, John K., 211*n*23

Illingworth, Patricia, 169, 191*n*25, 211*n*25

Immaculate infection, 89

Immigration: Ellis Island, 129; Emma Lazarus, 130; entitlement to, 141, 142; estimates of immigrants with HIV, 133, 134, 140; estimating costs of immigrants, 7, 130, 135–137, 140; history of law on, 129, 130; and homosexuality, 140, 141, 207*n*40; medical barriers to, 129, 131, 164; nativist concerns about, 129; policy on HIV, 7, 129, 130, 133; politics of, 109–110, 131–133, 140, 142–143, 164; protecting public health, 130–132, 133, 135; xenophobia, 130, 135, 138–140. *See also* Emigration

Immigration and Naturalization Service, 131

Imperial War Graves Commission, 64

India, 23

Informed consent: consistency of, 102, 107; disclosure of risks, 93, 94*ff*, 105; in health care relations, 94, 99; possibility of, 95*ff*. *See also* Health care relations

Institute of Medicine, 168, 211*n*22

Insurance, right of employers to limit, 141, 154, 208*n*45, 209*n*11

Ireland, 25

Irish, views of as unfit citizens, 142

Jeffrey, 196*n*36

Johnson, Earvin "Magic," 69, 72, 73, 76, 79, 82, 121, 145, 146, 198*n*14

Jonas, Hans, 158, 210*n*27

Jones, James W., 201*n*26

Jonsen, Albert R., 175–176, 195*n*81, 209*n*13, 211*n*32, 212*n*34

Joseph, Stephen, 41

Justice, Department of, 131
"Just say no," 147, 153

Kass, Leon, 210*n*10
Kemp, Jack, 209*n*10
Kennedy, John F., 183, 187
Kevorkian, Jack, 49, 195*n*79
"Kissing doesn't kill," 113, 116, 123–124, 125, 162, 204*n*17
Kleiner, Dick, 200*n*1
Koch, Ed, 41
Kopelman, Loretta M., 212*n*39
Kramer, Larry, 28, 77, 168, 198*n*18; belief in a cure, 48, 50; *Reports from the Holocaust,* 193*n*2, 195*n*76
Krauthammer, Charles, 162, 163
Kübler-Ross, Elisabeth, 4

Landers, Ann, 89
Lange, J. M. A., et al., 203*n*16
Laughter, 62
Law, tort remedies for HIV exposure, 104*ff. See also* Court decisions; Health care relations; Immigration
Lazarus, Emma, 130
Leavitt, David, 195*n*2
Leavitt, Judith Walzer, 207*n*42
Leibowitch, Jacques, 190*n*5
LeMay, Martin C., 208*n*50
Lesbians, and past exclusionary immigration policy, 140, 141
Letter to the editor. See *New England Journal of Medicine*
Liberace, 69, 78, 199*n*29
Libertarians, 174, 208*n*2
Life, 84, 200*n*10
Li Peng, 116
Longtime Companion: criticism of, 26, 192*n*52; narrative dissolution of time, 25–27
Love Alone. See Paul Monette
Lucas, Craig, 26
Ludlam, Charles, founder of the Ridiculous Theater, 56

MacIntyre, Alasdair, 176
"Magic bullet," 36, 41
Maingot, Anthony P., 207*n*41
Malone, looking for love, 54
Mann, Jonathan, 110, 204*n*2
Manzoni, Alessandro, 190*n*3

Marcel, Gabriel, 63
Marrou, Andre, 208*n*2
Marsden, P. D., 206*n*24
Mason, Belinda, member of National Commission on AIDS and self-described Tupperware housewife, 69
Matthews, Eric, 202*n*33
Maupin, Armistead, 195*n*2
McCauley, Stephen, 195*n*2
McKinney, Stuart, 69, 77–78
Medical Journal of Australia, 112, 204*n*9
Medicine: cures for homosexuality, 33; gay presence in, 32, 35; and homophobia, 29, 34–36; iatrogenic effects, 30*ff,* 44; limitations of, 38, 41, 43*ff;* orthodox, 39, 42. *See also* Cure; Health care relations; Research methods; Treatment
Mercitron, 49
Michael, went to Cornell, 56
Mickler, Ernie, author of *White Trash Cooking,* 55, 64
Military, bar on gay men and lesbians, 2, 200*n*11
Miller, James: "AIDS in the Novel," 13, 26, 191*n*13, 192*n*51, 206*n*26; *Passion of Michel Foucault,* 194*n*47, 198*n*19
Misogyny, 79
Mohr, Richard D., 8, 21, 169, 196*n*5, 200*n*11, 201*n*21, 211*n*24
Monette, Paul, 199*n*25; *Afterlife,* 37; *Borrowed Time,* 29*ff,* 58–59, 66; commitment to AIDS cure, 48; *Love Alone,* 58, 196*n*22; relation with Roger Horwitz, 30*ff,* 58–59, 64
Morbidity and Mortality Weekly Report, 33, 183, 187, 212*n*1
Murphy, Timothy F., 189*n*6, 192*n*49, 193*n*9, 193*n*18, 194*n*44, 198*n*19, 201*n*26, 204*n*15, 206*n*20, 212*n*33
Musto, David, 207*n*31, 207*n*39
Muzil. *See* Michel Foucault
The Myth of Heterosexual AIDS. See Michael Fumento

Names Project Memorial Quilt, 5, 60–61, 65, 150
National Commission on AIDS, 69, 130, 168

National Research Council, 49, 144, 156*ff*; authorship of report, 156; criticized, 157–160; description of epidemic, 156; description of social effects, 7, 156–157
Nativism, 129, 140. *See also* Emigration; Immigration
Navarre, Max, 201*n*26
Needle-exchange programs, 170
Needle-stick injuries, 82
New England Journal of Medicine: on celebrity disclosure, 70; letter to the editor, 69*ff*; views on physician responsibility, 75, 76
Nietzsche, Friedrich, 3, 4, 189*n*5
Nights in Aruba. See Andrew Holleran
North, David S., 207*n*29
Novak, William, 198*n*14
Novick, Alvin, 211*n*30
Nunokawa, Jeff, 64, 204*n*13
Nureyev, Rudolf, 78, 199*n*25

O., host par excellence, 56
Obituaries, 52*ff*, 59–60, 62–63
Office of Technology Assessment, 168
Orange County, California, 69
Orentlicher, David, 203*n*18
Original position. *See* John Rawls
Osborn, June, 130

Parran, Thomas, 206*n*19, 207*n*33
Pascal, Blaise, 26
Passions of the Cut Sleeve. See Bret Hinsch
Patient-physician relation. *See* Health care relations
Patient Self Determination Act, 49, 195*n*78
Patient Zero. *See* Gaetan Dugas
Peabody, Barbara, 54, 58
Pensées. See Blaise Pascal
Perkins, Anthony, 69, 78
Perot, Ross, 7, 144, 146, 149–151
Perrow, Charles, 168, 205*n*21, 211*n*18
Peters, Fritz, 195*n*1
Physicians: recruitment of celebrities to fight AIDS, *see* Celebrities; responsibility to disclose HIV/AIDS diagnoses, *see* Health care relations
Pierce, Christine, 212*n*39
Placebo effect, 45, 47–48
The Plague. See Albert Camus

The Plague (Die Seuche). See Peter Zingler
Plant, Richard, 204*n*12
Poersch, Enno, 197*n*42
Poirier, Suzanne, 192*n*49, 193*n*9, 198*n*19, 201*n*26, 204*n*15, 212*n*15
Presidential Commission on the Human Immunodeficiency Virus Epidemic, 158, 168, 172, 211*n*22
Presidential debate, 1992. *See* George Bush; Bill Clinton; Ross Perot
President's Task Force on Regulatory Relief, 148
Price, Monroe, 11, 20, 190*n*7–8; images of the future, 12, 20
Privacy: blurring distinction between public and private, 75, 106, 203*n*23; right to, 75
Private Acts, Social Consequences. See Ronald Bayer
Professor Zero, 109, 203*n*1
Promiscuity, as social artifact, 169, 170, 191*n*25
Proportional theory of resource provision. *See* Resource allocation
Public health: efforts to protect, 70, 76, 80, 133–135; threats to, 132–133, 135, 141
PWAs (Persons with AIDS): and activism, 48, 50, 89; as AIDS researchers, 29, 37, 48–49, 50; as experimental subjects, 29*ff*, 48–49; given voice, 56, 209*n*8; obituaries of, 52*ff*; representations of, 56; responsibilities of, 180; standing relative to resource allocation, 177–180; views on illness, 89, 193*n*27; visibility, 209*n*8

Quarantine: of Haitians with HIV, 138*ff*; symbolic purposes, 139

Ramsey, Paul, 176
Rawls, John: arguments from the original position, 102, 106–107, 178; contractarianism, 178–180; significance of the difference principle for PWAs, 178–179; *A Theory of Justice*, 102. *See also* Resource allocation

Reagan, Nancy, 147
Reagan, Ronald, 153, 205*n*1–2, 209*n*10
Reed, Robert, 78, 199*n*23
Religion and AIDS, 3, 4, 158, 167
Renal disease, 169
René, Norman, 26
Republican National Convention. *See* George Bush; Bill Clinton; Ross Perot
Research methods: conflicts between subjects and researchers, 45; favoritism in, 45, 46, 162; placebo effect, 45, 47–48
Resource allocation: AIDS spending, 2, 40–41, 137–148; criticism of AIDS spending, 148, 162, 163; determination of standards for, 165, 173*ff*; equalitarian theory of, 174; meritocratic theory of, 174–175; perfect and imperfect duties, 179–180; priority for AIDS, 7–8, 168–169, 171, 176, 177–178, 180–181; significance of voluntary risk, 147, 164, 165–166, 180; social obligations for, 160–161; utilitarian theory of, 173–174
Rider, Ines, 196*n*20
Rieux, Dr., 186
Robinson, Max, 78
Rogers, David E., 157, 197*n*8
Rolston, Adam, 113
Royko, Mike, 162
Ruddick, Paul, 196*n*36
Ruedy, J., et al., 211*n*19
Ruppelt, Patricia, 196*n*20
Ruskin, Cindy, 196*n*34
Russo, Vito, 48

St. Patrick's Cathedral, 146, 148–149, 208*n*6. *See also* Activism; ACT UP
Salk, Jonas, 45
Sande, Merle, 211*n*16
Sartre, Jean-Paul, 208*n*49
Schwartz, M. Roy, 197*n*8
Science, its authority, 24
The Screaming Room. See Barbara Peabody
Secretary for Health and Human Services. *See* Louis W. Sullivan

Selver, Veronica, 212*n*4
Die Seuche. See Peter Zingler
Sexual orientation therapy, 33, 193*n*18–19
Shadow in the Land. See William E. Dannemeyer
Shattered Mirrors. See Monroe Price
Shilts, Randy: on bathhouse closure, 15; characterization of Patient Zero, 11–19; disclosure of own diagnoses, 78; on gays and lesbians in the military, 200*n*11; on Kimberly Bergalis, 202*n*33
Siegler, Marc, 198*n*10
"Silence = Death," 86, 113
Smallpox, 171, 211*n*27
The Social Impact of AIDS in the United States. See National Research Council
Socrates, 187
Solomon, Robert, 197*n*39
"So many men, so little time," 15
Somerville, Margaret, 133, 135–136, 139, 206*n*26, 207*n*38
Sontag, Susan, 164
Spiers, Herbert R., 211*n*29
"Spread of AIDS," 3, 18, 27
Stambolian, George, 56
Statue of Liberty, 130
Stoddard, Thomas B., 89
Stryker, Jeff, 195*n*81, 209*n*13
Supererogatory moral duties, 170–171
Suramin, experimental drug, 32
Sutherland, drag queen, 54
Syphilis, 186, 206*n*19, 211*n*6

Taylor, Elizabeth, 77
Testimony: defined, 53, 57–58, 63, 65–66; and elegiac art, 5, 53*ff*, 57; purposes of, 6, 53, 57*ff*; worth of, 5–6, 57, 63
Testing. *See* HIV testing
Thailand, 23
Thanksgiving. See Elizabeth Cox
Time, narrative dissolution of. See *Long-time Companion*
Toga candida, 161
To the Friend Who Did Not Save My Life. See Hervé Guibert
Treatments for AIDS: effects of on PWAs, 29; orthodox, 38, 49; unorthodox, 28, 38–41, 44–45.

See also AZT; Cure; Research methods
Tuberculosis, 87
Tupperware housewife. *See* Belinda Mason
Tuskegee syphilis experiment, 33

University of Illinois at Chicago: Hospital and Clinics Ad Hoc Committee on HIV/HBV, 108–109, 120–121; Masters of Health Professions Education degree, 108
Unorthodox medicine, 38–41, 44–45
Utilitarian theory of resource provision. *See* Resource allocation

Vaccines, 38, 43*ff*, 45–47
VandeVeer, Donald, 212*n*39
Vaux, Kenneth L., 189*n*8
Veatch, Robert, 170, 211*n*26
Veil of Ignorance. *See* John Rawls
Victims of AIDS: analysis of term, 89, 90, 147, 201*n*23; "innocent victims," 84, 86, 89, 90; use of term, 89, 111, 147–148, 204*n*6. *See also* Kimberly Bergalis
Virginity, kinds and moral meanings of, 90
VonLehn, Peter, aspired to career in opera, 54, 64
Voodoo, 138, 207*n*32

Watney, Simon, 192*n*1
Westminster Abbey, 64
What You Can Do to Avoid AIDS. See Earvin "Magic" Johnson
White, Ryan, 69, 76, 82, 84, 197*n*4
White Trash Cooking. See Ernie Mickler
Wojnarowicz, David: "Living Close to the Knives," 38*ff*; "X Rays from Hell," 40–41
Wolf, Peter, 35
Women, 171; as harbingers of AIDS, 85–86; as research subjects, 42, 194. *See also* Kimberly Bergalis
World Health Organization, 211*n*27
Worth, Dooley, 210*n*12

Xenophobia: and China, 111, 121–122; and Haiti, 138*ff*; nativism, 129, 140. *See also* Immigration

Yale Law Project, 202*n*20
Yeomans, Beryl June, 64
Yeomans, Laura Rose, 64
Yeomans, George Alfred, 64
Young, Frank, 41
Young, James Harvey, 189*n*4, 194*n*37, 208*n*5

Zeldis, Nancy, 205*n*5
Zemke, Deborah, 196*n*34
Zingler, Peter, dystopia novelist, 25

Designer: U.C. Press Staff
Compositor: Braun-Brumfield, Inc.
Text: 10/13 Galliard
Display: Galliard
Printer: Braun-Brumfield, Inc.
Binder: Braun-Brumfield, Inc.